Right Now!

Practical Strategies for Anxiety, Depression, and Suicidal Thinking

Praise for *Right Now!*

I absolutely love Suzanne Oliver's new book, *Right Now! Practical Strategies for Anxiety, Depression, and Suicidal Thinking*. I have learned so much from her book and was easily able to identify with her and appreciate the information that she so freely shares. Each section flows easily into the next, and her writing is clear and concise, which in turn does not overwhelm the reader. I especially enjoyed the way in which she has given alternative suggestions and resources since, as she mentions, some protocols may not work for some individuals. Suzanne's book is for anyone and loved ones who have struggled with mental illness and suicide, leaving the reader educated and inspired that there is hope.

—Jessica Garcia, RMT, KRMT, ACM, Angel Healer

Right Now! Practical Strategies for Anxiety, Depression, and Suicidal Thinking is an insightful and compassionate guide to suicide prevention and overall wellness. Blending practical strategies with emotional support, this book emphasizes the importance of mental, physical, and spiritual well-being in navigating life's challenges. Through a holistic approach, it offers tools for self-care, resilience, and personal growth, making it a valuable resource for those struggling or supporting others in crisis. With its uplifting tone and actionable advice, this book serves as both a prevention tool and a roadmap to a happier, more balanced life.

—Judy Drilling, University of Phoenix, Professor of Psychology

A Lifeline for Those in Darkness

This book is a **must-read** for anyone struggling with **anxiety, depression, or suicidal thoughts**—it truly has the power to **save lives.** The author, having endured the unimaginable pain or losing both her son and husband to suicide, has turned her personal tragedy into a **beacon of hope** for others.

With profound compassion and unwavering strength, she shares her journey, offering not just words or comfort but also **practical tools and invaluable resources** to guide those in crisis toward healing. Her **holistic mind–body–spirit approach** ensures that readers receive well-rounded support, addressing both emotional wounds and deeper spiritual aspects of recovery.

This book is more than a memoir; it is a roadmap to resilience, a testament to the human spirit, and a **lifeline** for anyone who feels lost in the darkness. This book could make all the difference if you or someone you love is struggling. **Highly recommended.**

—Author Rev. Janette Freeman, PhD

This book is a heartfelt, well-researched guide for anyone desiring more health in mind, body, or spirit; it's a go-to reference with techniques to help relieve anxiety and depression in themselves or a loved one. Excellent!

—Jackie Taggart, Special Education Teacher,
Science of Mind Practitioner

Right Now!

Practical Strategies for Anxiety, Depression, and Suicidal Thinking

Suzanne K. Oliver

Mind-Body-Spirit Press
Fresno, California

The information contained in this book is based on current research and the author has made every effort to ensure the information is complete and accurate. The suggestions in this book are not a replacement for medical advice. The author is not liable for any injury or damage allegedly arising from these suggestions. Always consult with your healthcare provider before starting any medical regimen, dietary suggestions, or spiritual practices.

This book is dedicated to Josh—my son who left this Earthly life too young. Your suffering will be an inspiration to others—to focus on their total well-being—mind, body, and spirit. Until we meet again. I love you forever.

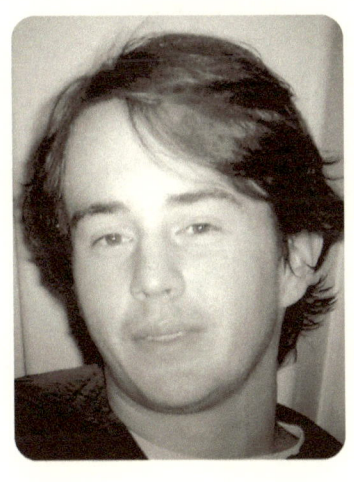

Table of Contents

~ I ~
A Message from the Author

The ideas presented in this book are based on my passion for helping families and friends who have loved ones with anxiety, depression, and/or suicidal thoughts. My initial thought was that if I can help even one person struggling with thoughts of suicide, this book will have been worth the effort. However, since completing this book my thoughts have changed; I want to help as many people as I can, not just one. I don't want anyone else to experience the pain of losing someone they love to suicide.

In 2007, my oldest son, Josh, took his own life at age 21. He had been suffering from depression and anxiety for many years. When he was a young teenager, my husband and I took him to counseling but it didn't help because there was no focus on what the problem was. He became much more depressed in high school and refused to go to school. He completed an online program, but it was difficult because he was not motivated to do his assignments. I worked full time but would sit with him to complete his lessons when I got home each day. It was very difficult for everyone.

After Josh graduated, he held different jobs but was still depressed and anxious. The only thing he really enjoyed was playing the online game World of Warcraft. He ended up quitting his job and staying home to play his game. We would often talk to him about how he was feeling and he finally told us one day that he didn't want to live. As you can imagine, we were terrified. We went with him to see his general practitioner and Josh told the doctor that he was having thoughts of suicide. She was very concerned and said he needed a psychiatric evaluation. We immediately got on the phone and contacted the doctors she recommended but none were available for several months.

Finally, we found a doctor who had an opening within the month. I didn't know anything about mental health issues at the time, so I deferred to my husband who was in the medical field. I wish I had known then what I do now; the practices discussed in this book could have led to a very different outcome.

Within minutes, the psychiatrist determined that Josh had bipolar disorder. This devasted Josh—he thought he was doomed to feel that way the rest of his life. Josh was 21 and because of HIPAA laws the doctor was unable to disclose Josh's treatment and their discussions without his permission. Josh authorized the doctor to discuss everything with us, but after he took his own life, we discovered the doctor did not tell us everything. In his sessions, Josh revealed three different occasions that he tried to take his life. The doctor did not share this with us but immediately put Josh on antidepressant and antianxiety medications.

Josh began taking the medications and was told to increase the antidepressant dose until he reached the therapeutic level—standard procedure. After a week, he got worse. We asked the doctor what we should do but were told that Josh needed to reach the therapeutic dosage; he had to continue increasing it. We also spoke to the pharmacist at our local pharmacy and were told the same thing. We trusted that these professionals knew what they were talking about since they were the "experts."

Another week went by, and Josh continued to get worse. Again, we called the doctor and were told the same thing. When we called the third time, the doctor did not answer so we left a desperate message. The next day, our internet went out and Josh was unable to play World of Warcraft, the only thing he could do. The internet provider said they could not fix the problem for five days. After Josh heard this, he got even worse. The doctor still had not returned our calls two days later, but his dad and I had to go to work. At around 3 p.m. that day, I received the worst phone call any parent could ever get; one of my sons returned from school and found his brother.

Unfortunately, the tragedy did not end there. My two younger sons, my husband, and I were all deeply affected. We went to family counseling, which was very painful. My husband blamed himself for Josh's mental illness since he also had suffered from depression his whole life. I feel the counseling helped tremendously, but for two years I was sleepwalking through life. I couldn't rest without antianxiety meds and sleeping pills, making it nearly impossible to function the next day. I started reading books about suicide, near-death experiences, spirit communications, and anything I could find to comfort me, to feel that Josh was okay in the spirit realm. This led me to a New Thought church that gave me enormous comfort. I studied the principles and became a practitioner of Science of Mind (explained later) that helped me shift my thinking.

In 2011, my husband took his own life, and our family was devastated once more. I struggled again emotionally, but being very involved in my church and using the practices I had learned helped. I became interested in helping other people shift their thinking, but I had no idea how to do it; I was learning many strategies to help shift energy and thinking, but depressed people are not motivated to help themselves. So, over 15 years after Josh's death, I collected material from any source that could benefit mental health. I would learn something helpful, research it, then put it in my file. I wasn't sure how I could distribute the information to help people, but I trusted that when the time was right, I would know what direction to go.

In 2024, I realized that with a bit more research on preventing suicide, I could write a book. This book is an organized collection of that information I've learned along the way, plus current research. It has become apparent that helping someone with a mental illness requires a holistic approach that includes all aspects of life: mind, body, and spirit. If I'd had the compilation of resources that you now hold in your hand, I may have been able to help Josh. With the strategies and practices in this book, you will be better informed about mental illness and how to help your loved one.

DISCLAIMER: The author is not a mental health expert and nothing in this book should be construed as advice. The information contained in this book is based on current research and the author has made every effort to ensure it is complete and accurate; the author is not liable for any injury or damage allegedly arising from these suggestions. Consult a healthcare provider for a personalized plan of action.

~ II ~
Warning Signs of Suicide and Resources

Although the world is full of suffering,
it is also full of the overcoming of it.
—Helen Keller

There are many warning signs that indicate that a person is thinking about suicide. One line of thought that has bothered me over the years is that a person who talks about suicide will not follow through with it. I can speak from experience that this is not always the case; my son told us he didn't want to live, and he did take his own life. Not everyone expresses their feelings and that's why it is important to recognize warning signs and take *immediate* action.

A visual of some warning signs to note is at suicideispreventable. org and for teens, includes the following: increased alcohol and drug use, talking about wanting to die, uncontrolled anger, reckless behavior, changes in sleep, feeling hopeless, desperate, or trapped, having no sense of purpose, putting affairs in order, giving their possessions away, anxiety or agitation, sudden mood changes, withdrawal, and talking about being a burden to others. For adults, the warning signs also include seeking methods for self-harm such as searching online or obtaining a gun and talking about feeling hopeless or having no reason to live. The Cleveland Clinic[1] states other warning signs to be aware of - a person not finding joy in life, sudden calmness, and writing a note.

It is important recognize these symptoms because suicide is one of the leading causes of death in the United States. The statistics are alarming; every 11 minutes someone dies by suicide. The Cleveland Clinic breaks this down by age.

- Ages 10–14 Second leading cause of death
- Ages 15–24: Third leading cause of death
- Ages 25-34: Second leading cause of death
- Ages 35–44: Fourth leading cause of death

Certain groups of people are more at risk than others: Alaskan Native, incarcerated, LGBTQIA+, Indigenous, isolated, non-Hispanic White, male, migrant or refugee, 65+ years, veteran, victim of violence of abuse, and victim of war or natural disaster.

Concerns should never be taken lightly but you need to know where to get help. Below is a list of resources for a starting point but remember that the primary care physician should also be included.

The 988 Suicide and Crisis Lifeline, formally The National Suicide Prevention Lifeline, is a 24-hour-a-day, seven-day-a-week phone number for anyone feeling suicidal or for someone who has thoughts of harming others, anxiety, issues related to gender identity, overwhelming feelings regarding finances, food, and housing, being all alone and needing to talk to someone, and feelings of being in a crisis. You can also call this number for advice if you have concerns about a loved one. When a person calls 988, they are connected to a trained counselor who can provide emotional support and share relevant resources. There is also a text feature option for those who prefer that method of communication. Calling or texting 988 is free and confidential.

Suicide hotlines are found in every country and are listed on The International Association for Suicide Prevention website.[2] This website also has numbers to call or text and numbers for specific groups of people, such as veterans, LGBTQ+, and others. Each state's mental health resources can be found with a simple Google search. A trained counselor at Crisis Text Line is available 24/7 by texting a message to 741741. Their vision is "an empathetic world where nobody feels alone."[3]

Children/youths and students:

- Hey Sam for youth: 439726

- Youth Hotline: 839963 or 877-968-8491

- Teen Line: 839863 or 800-852-8336

- Trevor Lifeline for LGBTQ+ youth: 678678 or 866-488-7386

- Safe Place TXT 4 Help for youth and children: 44357

- National Grad Crisis Line: 877-472-3457

Deaf/hard of hearing

- SAMHSA's National Hotline: 435748 or 800-662-4357

LGBTQ+

- Trevor Lifeline for LGBTQ+ and youth: 678678 or 866-488-7386

- LGBT National Hotline for LGBTQ+: 888-843-4564

- LGBT National Senior Helpline for LGBT+ and seniors: 888-234-7243

- LGBT National Coming Out Support Hotline for LGBTQ+: 888-688-5428

Veterans

- Veterans Crisis Line: 838255
- Centerstone Military Services for Veterans: 866-781-8010

Crisis lifelines for everyone:

- Physician Support Line: 888-409-0141
- Childhelp's Courage First Athlete Helpline: 888-279-1026
- National Alliance on Mental Illness (NAMI): 62640 or 800-950-6264
- SAMHSA's National Hotline: 435748 or 800-662-4357
- National Parent and Youth Hotline: call or text 855-427-2736
- BlackLine: 800-604-5841
- Su Familia: 866-783-2645

To start a conversation with someone who is suicidal, visit the website suicideispreventable.org. The basic steps are:

1. Start the conversation.
2. Listen, express concern, reassurance.
3. Create a safety plan.
4. Get help.

Things you should not say:

- You're not thinking about suicide, are you?
- Fine! If you want to be selfish and kill yourself, then go right ahead! See if I care.
- Don't worry, I won't tell anyone. Your secret is safe with me.

From the research I've done and the experiences I've had, it's vitally important to communicate effectively with someone who is suicidal. A national program that teaches how to talk to someone who is suicidal is the QPR Institute[4] that offers a 90-minute training program for those who are interested in learning this technique. QPR stands for Question, Persuade, Refer. I'm sure there are other resources available, but the ones discussed above are a good place to start. It's crucial to act immediately if you are concerned that someone might harm themself.

Suggestion: If you are concerned that a person is thinking about suicide, contact appropriate resources and ensure your loved one has the number in their phone. Make an appointment with their primary care physician. Educate yourself on how to effectively talk to that person.

~ III ~
About This Book

We are not human beings having a spiritual experience;
we are spiritual beings having a human experience.
—Pierre Teilhard de Chardin

We are spiritual beings first because we existed in spiritual form before we were born into the physical world. Being spiritual does not mean religious; it means our personal relationship with God. If we look at life this way, healing is a soul-centered approach. That is why we need to focus on healing spiritually along with the body and mind. The three are all interconnected and that is why the focus of this book is to treat someone with anxiety, depression, and/or suicidal thinking by focusing on all three aspects of life.

This book is addressed to loved ones who have someone struggling with anxiety, depression, and/or suicidal thinking because, oftentimes, the person experiencing these emotions is unable to help themselves. That doesn't mean that depressed or anxious people cannot help themselves, but someone else may need to help them initiate healing practices.

There are three sections of this book: one for the mind, one for the body, and one for the spirit. Although three distinct sections, all are interconnected; when healing occurs in one area, it positively affects the other areas. I recommend reading the introduction to each section first, then look at all the chapters included and read the chapters that resonate with you first. Then, go back and read the other chapters. Some of the practices in each section are easy to implement while others are much more intensive.

I believe that counseling is a critical part of the treatment plan for lasting change in thinking and behavior. I am not a doctor—the suggestions I make are just that, *suggestions*; discuss a course of action with your doctor or psychologist. A person talking about suicide should never be taken lightly. The suicide lifeline 988 is available 24 hours a day, seven days a week in English and Spanish. This number can be called or texted.

My goal in writing this book is to give people options and ideas to implement when a loved one is suicidal, because I was not given that kind of support when my son told me he wanted to die. I was just told he needed to see a psychiatrist. While seeing a psychiatrist was good advice, it was not enough for him. Medication alone does not address underlying problems; it just covers up the symptoms in most cases. By addressing all aspects of life—mind, body, and spirit—the focus on is healing, not covering up.

> **Suggestion:** Read the introduction to each section first, then read the chapters that resonate with you. Read the remainder of the book in any order.

~ IV ~
Introduction: Mind

Folks are usually about as happy as they make their minds up to be.
—Abraham Lincoln

I feel this is the most important part of the book because even when we incorporate our body and our spirit into healing, the brain is the organ that controls and coordinates our actions and reactions. That is why I believe finding a reputable psychotherapist is critical when treating anxiety and depression. Working with a therapist, patients learn to change problematic thinking and feelings. I have found that our beliefs are immensely powerful; if we think something will work, it will. This is called the placebo effect. Many studies have been done on the placebo effect, which basically means that when a person believes a treatment will work, it will. Dr. Wayne W. Dyer wrote an entire book on this subject called *You'll See It When You Believe It*[5] in which he discusses how we need to believe something to be true before it does become true. I have practiced this belief for years and have seen the results of believing something to be true, even while having symptoms, and it does become true.

The Biology of Belief[6] by stem cell biologist and epigenetics expert Bruce H. Lipton, PhD, says that our mind has the power to change our cells; in contrast to doctors who believe our genes determine our health, Lipton theorizes that our perception of the environment determines our health, not the other way around.

For some people experiencing severe depression, psychotherapy and/or medications are not enough. This is known as treatment-resistant depression, and you'll find other options to consider in this chapter. There is also a section on brain imaging, a test in which malfunctioning areas of the brain are pinpointed so treatment can be focused on those areas.

A variety of practices that can help shift thinking are discussed in this section and include practicing gratitude, kindness, positive self-affirmations, forgiveness, and being around positive people.

The chapter on pharmaceuticals discusses how medications are often used in treating anxiety and depression. As you read this section, take notes so you can discuss the options with your physician. The last few chapters discuss things that can increase anxiety and depression such as social media, the news, too much TV, and drug and alcohol use.

> **Suggestion:** Have regular appointments with a reputable psychotherapist. Practice gratitude, forgiveness, kindness, self-affirmations, and interact with positive people. Avoid or limit social media, the news, and too much TV. Avoid drugs and alcohol altogether.

1

......

Psychological Counseling
(Psychotherapy)

A good counselor can be the guiding light
that helps you navigate through the darkest storms.
—Unknown

Finding a psychotherapist to work with is crucial for someone who is suicidal. This may take some time; the first one might not be a good fit. The executive director of counseling and support services at Hinds Hospice says someone who thinks that therapy is not for them may simply not have met the right counselor.[7] If the counselor does not seem like a good fit, keep trying until there is a connection and the person feels comfortable with the professional.

A psychotherapist, whether a psychiatrist, psychologist, or a mental health professional—can help individuals learn strategies to overcome depression according to the Mayo Clinic.[8] Below are some therapies and a brief description of each.

1. **Cognitive behavioral therapy (CBT):** The American Psychological Association (APA)[9] states "CBT is a form of psychological treatment that has been demonstrated to be effective for a range of problems including depression, anxiety disorders, alcohol and drug use problems, marital problems, eating disorders, and severe mental illness." Many research studies to

determine the effectiveness of CBT have demonstrated that CBT is "as effective or more effective as other forms of psychological therapy or psychiatric medications." CBT is based on three core principles according to the APA:

a. Psychological problems are based, in part, on faulty or unhelpful ways of thinking.

b. Psychological problems are based, in part, on learned patterns of unhelpful behavior.

c. People suffering from psychological problems can learn better ways of coping with them, thereby relieving their symptoms and becoming more effective in their lives.

2. **Eye movement desensitization and reprocessing (EMDR):** EMDR Institute[10] states "EMDR is a psychotherapy that enables people to heal from the symptoms and emotional distress that are the result of disturbing life experiences." EMDR was founded in 1987 by Dr. Francine Shapiro and is widely used for treating severe emotional pain that previously took years of psychological therapy to treat. To find a therapist trained in EMDR go to emdr.com and enter your location.

3. **Acceptance and commitment therapy:** This is a form of CBT that teaches engagement in positive behaviors despite negative thoughts and emotions.

4. **Personal psychotherapy:** Working one-on-one with a trained mental health professional for individual counseling.

5. **Interpersonal therapy (IPT):** Short-term psychotherapy focused on improving mental health symptoms by improving relationships. This therapy is helpful for anxiety, depression, mood disorders (bipolar and dysthymic disorders), and PTSD (post-traumatic stress disorder)

6. **Family or marital therapy:** This therapy is for working out stressful issues with family members or a spouse.

7. **Dialectical behavior therapy:** DBT is a type of talk therapy (psychotherapy) based on CBT, but it's specially adapted for people who experience emotions very intensely." The focus is on helping people accept their lives and their behaviors.[11]

8. **Group psychotherapy:** Psychotherapist-run group meetings for people with depression.

9. **Mindfulness:** Being mindful of thoughts and feelings without judging them.

10. **Behavioral activation:** A gradual approach to decrease avoidance and isolation and increase involvement in activities once enjoyed.

Here are some other effective therapies.

1. **Analytical psychotherapy:** Focuses on past experiences with the aim of finding possible psychological causes.

2. **Depth psychotherapy:** Similar to analytical psychotherapy but focuses more on current conflicts.

3. **Systematic therapy:** Includes the family—helping them communicate better and giving each other more support.

Cognitive behavioral therapy is also effective in treating anxiety disorders. The APA[12] lists types of anxiety disorders:

1. **Generalized anxiety disorder:** Persistent feelings of worry.

2. **Panic disorder:** Recurring panic attacks.

3. **Phobias:** An intense fear of certain objects or situations.

4. **Social anxiety disorder:** The fear of social situations because of feeling self-conscious or worrying that someone will judge them.

5. **Obsessive-compulsive disorder (OCD):** Obsessing on certain thoughts, routines, or rituals.

6. **PTSD:** Flashbacks or nightmares of a trauma. An additional resource for PTSD is a stellate ganglion block, which is a nerve that controls our fight-or-flight response. (Visit nimh.nih.gov for more information.)

There is one more form of psychotherapy not listed above that the Cleveland Clinic states can treat many mental health conditions such as depression, panic attacks, phobias, PTSD, and stress or anxiety—hypnotherapy.[13] While effective for many conditions, there are risks with this therapy and it is not recommended for people suffering from delusions, hallucinations, or other psychotic conditions. Consult with your doctor before starting such a treatment.

Mental health workers suggest additional practices, such as peer support groups, where people who have lived through the experience of suicide can offer support to others.

If an individual does not respond to either medications or psychotherapy, they are likely to have treatment-resistant depression. Options for this condition are discussed in the next chapter.

> **Suggestion:** Discuss the available treatment options with a reputable psychotherapist.

2

....

Treatment-Resistant Depression

Up to 33% of people with depression don't respond
to multiple kinds of conventional antidepressants.
—Johns Hopkins Medicine[14]

If antidepressants, counseling, and/or more holistic approaches have not been successful in treating depression, it might be that you are dealing with treatment-resistant depression. An abstract from the National Library of Medicine (NLM) said that while there is no consensus definition of treatment-resistant depression (TRD), the most used is from the United States Food and Drug Administration (FDA) and the European Medicine Agency (EMA) which describes it as "inadequate response to a minimum of two antidepressants despite adequacy of the treatment trial and adherence to treatment."[15] As stated in the quote above, over 30% of those suffering from depression meet these criteria.

The Mayo Clinic[16] recommends other options to discuss with your doctor if TRD has been determined.

1. **Repetitive transcranial magnetic stimulation (rTMS):** As the name suggests, this approach uses magnets to stimulate the nerve cells and improve the symptoms of depression.

2. **Ketamine:** A controversial treatment administered intravenously at a physician's office. This treatment can have significant side effects; certain people should not use it.

3. **Electroconvulsive therapy (ECT):** Brief seizures are induced by using electricity while the subject is sleeping. ECT changes the brain chemistry to reverse symptoms of major depression. Side effects are temporary confusion and memory loss.

4. **Vagus nerve stimulation (VNS):** A device implanted in the chest connects with the vagus nerve to stimulate it with an electrical signal. This treatment can be tried if ECT and rTMS have not been successful.

Johns Hopkins Medicine recommends additional options:

1. **Deep brain stimulation (DBS):** A surgical procedure places a small device under the collarbone that connects to wires in the brain.

2. **Psilocybin:** Derived from a hallucinogenic mushroom, this drug, similar to LSD, is given in a controlled environment alongside psychotherapy. As of early 2025, it was not FDA-approved but was being evaluated for its effects on depression.

The Cleveland Clinic also has recommendations for treatment-resistant depression:

1. **Esketamine nasal spray:** FDA approved this derivative of ketamine in 2019 to be used in conjunction with an oral antidepressant. Following treatment, a person must be monitored by a health care provider for two hours. It can provide remission from depression symptoms within this time.

2. **Quetiapine and olanzapine:** Affecting dopamine levels, these may improve depression symptoms.

3. **Aripiprazole and brexpiprazole:** Adjusts serotonin and norepinephrine levels, which may improve depression symptoms.

4. **Lithium:** FDA approved this only for depression associated with bipolar disorder.

One more treatment option, discussed briefly in chapter 1, especially for PTSD, is a *stellate ganglion block (SGB)*. Most people are not aware of this procedure because it is often used for pain management, but it is worth checking into because of the benefits for those suffering from PTSD, anxiety, and depression. The Cleveland Clinic defines an SGB as "an injection of anesthetic medication into a collection of nerves called the stellate ganglion."[17] Blocking these nerves in the neck controls the body's fight-or-flight response. This out-patient procedure performed by a pain specialist is usually about 30 minutes, followed by 40 minutes to an hour of observation. Not everyone has a stellate ganglion but 80% of the world's population does.

Dr. Jason Attaman[18] says that this block is effective 85% of the time but the Cleveland Clinic, which has been studying the effects on PTSD since 1990, states that there are mixed results on the effectiveness. As of early 2025, this procedure was not FDA approved but some healthcare providers still consider the SGB if other treatments have not been effective in reducing PTSD. The Cleveland Clinic lists a variety of possible short-term side effects including bruising or soreness at the injection site, drooping eyelids, red eyes, watery eyes, nasal stuffiness, hoarse voice, feeling of a lump in the throat, difficulty swallowing, and warmth or tingling in the arm or hand. While this seems like a lot of possible side effects, they are usually gone by the next day and experiencing them is a good sign because it means the injection was in the correct place. Rare but more serious side effects include infection, bleeding from a vascular puncture, damage to the vagus nerve, recurrent nerve or brachial plexus roots, pneumothorax, thyroid injury, esophageal and tracheal puncture, and transient Horner's Syndrome.

If an SGB is effective, the procedure may need to be repeated from two to ten times. A local pain specialist can help determine if this treatment is a possibility. Not all insurances cover SGB, so check into that also. Like all other treatments, it is important to continue psychotherapy and make other positive changes in your life discussed in this book.

Fortunately, other options are available if a person is not responding to standard treatments. It is also a good idea to get a second opinion from a specialist in depression.

Suggestion: A person who is not responding to treatment needs to talk to their doctor or psychiatrist about options for treatment-resistant depression.

3

Brain Imaging

With a better brain, EVERYTHING in your life is BETTER,
including your physical health, work, relationships, finances,
learning, energy, mood, and memory.
—Daniel G. Amen, MD[19]

Brain imaging can be useful in detecting certain neurological conditions, but in psychiatry, it is mainly used to rule out other medical conditions. I have learned that psychiatrists make a subjective diagnosis in which they interview the client and the family using the *Diagnostic and Statistical Manual of Mental Disorders* (DSM). On the other hand, brain imaging allows for an objective evaluation that takes the guess out of the root causes, as seen in the brain.

The quote above is from Daniel G. Amen, founder of the Amen Clinic, Inc. His approach is to use SPECT (single photon emission computer tomography) imaging of the brain. I have personal experience with the Amen Clinic. After my son died by suicide in 2007, one of my sons had an extremely hard time; terrible anxiety, panic attacks, and a whole list of problems, so in 2011, I took him to the Amen Clinic for an evaluation. I was extremely impressed by the process.

First, he had an interview with a trained outcome manager who asked about symptoms in four areas of his life: biological, psychological, social, and spiritual. This information was reviewed by one of the Amen Clinic physicians. After this, we went to one of the 11 clinics they hold throughout the United States, and he had a SPECT scan that measured the blood flow and activity in the brain. After the interview and evaluation of the SPECT scan results, the physician made a diagnosis. Alongside this report there were recommendations for blood work, specific medications/supplements, and psychotherapy to address the problems discovered in my son's brain. Each person's brain is different so what was recommended for him won't benefit someone else. Each treatment is individualized.

The Amen Clinic diagnoses and treats over 40 conditions, but the following list is specific to anxiety and depression.

1. Attention deficit disorder (ADD)
2. Anger issues, violent behavior, and IED
3. Anxiety
4. Bipolar disorder
5. Depression
6. Drugs and alcohol addiction
7. Mania and hypomania
8. Obsessive-compulsive disorder (OCD)
9. Panic disorder and panic attacks
10. Post-traumatic stress disorder (PTSD)
11. Postpartum depression
12. Psychosis and early psychosis
13. Seasonal affective disorder (SAD)
14. Self-harm
15. Sleep disorders
16. Stress
17. Suicidal thoughts and behavior
18. Treatment-resistant conditions

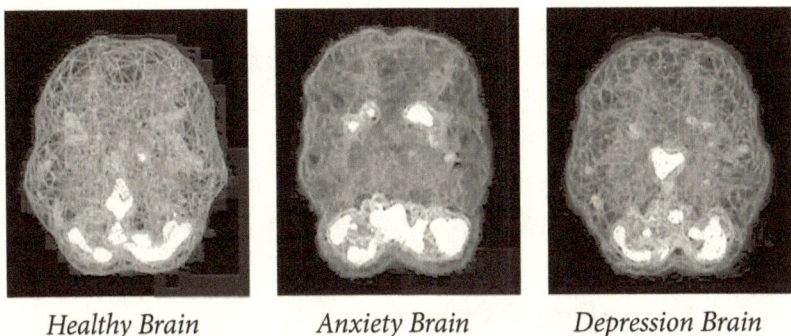

Healthy Brain   *Anxiety Brain*   *Depression Brain*

SPECT scans courtesy of the Amen Clinic

From the variety of conditions the Amen Clinic treats, it is evident that proper diagnosis is critical to effective treatment. While my son did not want to take the recommended medications or supplements, he did receive psychotherapy, as did I, and was able to overcome the anxiety and panic attacks. I experienced many of the same symptoms as my son and decided not to take medication but decided to take the supplements that were recommended for him (I wasn't on any medication, so I wasn't worried about negative side effects). After a couple of months, my anxiety had greatly improved, and I was able to function again. I have since stopped taking some of the supplements, but I continue to benefit from two of them.

Along with SPECT imaging, the Amen Clinic offers a variety of services, including telehealth and video therapy, psychiatric evaluations, supplement and medication management, memory rescue programs, concussion rescue programs, hyperbaric oxygen therapy, integrative medicine, psychotherapy, individual therapy, family therapy, hypnotherapy, cognitive behavior therapy, QEEG brain mapping, IV nutrition therapy, neurofeedback, hormone evaluation and replacement therapy, Irlen Syndrome screening, nutritional services, coaching, sports psychiatry program, EMDR therapy, integrative metronome training, forensic psychiatry, and neuroinflammatory intensive programs.

Dr. Daniel G. Amen has been a psychiatrist for over 30 years and is the founder of Change Your Brain Foundation.[20] He feels "the current state-of-the-art in psychiatry is unacceptable." On its website, he gives examples of scans done on parts of the body when there is a physical problem, but when the problem is in the brain, no scans are performed, which he finds unacceptable. His foundation has three purposes:

1. Provide innovative mental health/brain health services for people who cannot afford it.

2. Provide education on brain health to as many people as possible. We currently have a high school/college course in all 50 states and seven countries.

3. Conduct research dedicated to changing how psychiatric medicine is practiced by adding neuroimaging and natural ways to heal the brain.

Additional information is available on their website. The Amen Clinic does not accept medical insurance but facilitates a payment plan.

Suggestion: Discuss SPECT imaging with a psychiatrist/general practitioner to evaluate possible benefits.

4

Gratitude

Some people grumble that roses have thorns;
I am grateful that thorns have roses.
—Alphonse Karr

Practicing gratitude can have a positive effect on mental health because of the shift from negative to positive thoughts, which, according to several studies, reduces stress and anxiety. Benefits from practicing gratitude include strengthening relationships, improved sleep quality, higher levels of happiness and life satisfaction, reducing negative ruminations, promoting positive thinking, reducing cortisol (the stress hormone), promoting self-esteem and self-worth, and reducing depression.

Ashley J. Smith, a psychologist, professional speaker, and co-founder of Peak Mind: The Center for Psychological Strength, wrote an article for the Anxiety & Depression Association of America.[21] In it, Smith explains how gratitude relates to anxiety and depression; both are associated with negative thinking so focusing on gratitude can decrease anxiety, depression, and anger. She states that practicing gratitude helps individuals to recognize and value small aspects of life, which can enhance overall happiness and well-being. One treatment approach, habit reversal training (HRT), uses a competing response incompatible with the habit you are trying to break. The example she gives is a nailbiter who is trained to clasp their hands, impeding the habit. In the same way, being grateful is incompatible with negative thinkings, so it reduces the negative ruminations, worry, and complaining.

A study done by Dr. Joshua Brown and Dr. Joel Wong from Indiana University[22] showed the benefits of gratitude to our brain. Their study comprised 300 students at the university who sought counseling for anxiety and depression. The participants were divided into three groups: the first was asked to write one letter of gratitude to someone for three weeks, the second was to write about their negative life experiences, and the third was not asked to do any writing. Dr. Brown and Dr. Wong discovered "those who wrote gratitude letters reported significantly better mental health four weeks and 12 weeks after their writing exercises ended" and that practicing gratitude in conjunction with counseling was more beneficial than counseling alone. They also learned four additional components of gratitude:

1. Gratitude unshackles us from toxic emotions.

2. It helps even if it's not shared.

3. Its benefits take time.

4. It has lasting effects on the brain.

Not only does gratitude shift our thinking from negative to positive, but it also helps us attract what we want in life. This is accomplished through the law of attraction, a New Thought spiritual teaching that positive beliefs bring about positive experiences and negative beliefs bring about negative experiences. Although there is no scientific evidence to prove this, it is believed that our thoughts are "pure energy" and like thoughts attract like experiences. For example, if you have trouble sleeping but practice gratitude, you will be grateful for the one or two hours of uninterrupted sleep you do get. According to the law of attraction, as you focus on the quality of sleep you got, you would get more quality sleep. *The Magic* by Rhonda Byrne[23] explains how to practice gratitude and outlines a 28-day plan to incorporate it into your life. Below are just 10 ways[24] to become more grateful:

1. Gratitude journal: Write daily what you are grateful for.

2. Remember the bad to remind yourself how far you've come.

3. Ask yourself three questions: "What have I received from _____?" "What have I given to _____?" and "What trouble and difficulties have I caused?"

4. Share your gratitude with others; when someone does something you appreciate, express your gratitude with them.

5. Come to your senses as a way to appreciate being alive.

6. Use visual reminders as cues to trigger thoughts of gratitude.

7. Make a vow to practice gratitude; write it down and post it as a reminder.

8. Watch your language, focusing on good things others have done for you.

9. Go through the motions of smiling, saying "thank you," and writing letters of gratitude, which will trigger the emotion of gratitude more often.

10. Think outside the box. Look for creative situations to feel gratitude.

Calm.com lists 10 similar ways to incorporate gratitude into your life and you can download their app for guided meditations.[25]

1. Keep a gratitude journal.

2. Express gratitude to loved ones.

3. Practice gratitude meditations (YouTube has many guided meditations).

4. Gratitude jar: Write down what you are grateful for and put it in a jar.

5. Volunteer or give back.

6. Set gratitude alarms as a reminder.

7. Practice gratitude walks.

8. Say "thank you" more often.

9. Reflect on your challenges, focusing on how these challenges helped you grow.

10. Gratitude visualization: Vividly imagine things you're grateful for.

Suggestion: Choose at least one method of practicing gratitude from the lists above and incorporate it into your daily life.

5

·············

Kindness

How do we change the world? One random act of kindness at a time.
—Morgan Freeman

Kindness is important when it comes to a depressed person because, as explained in Chapter 25 on energy, a depressed person is vibrating at a low frequency, the level of shame in which their core belief is that they are not good enough, according to David Hawkins, MD, PhD. Kindness is much higher on David Hawkins' Map of Consciousness[26] as discussed in his book *Power vs Force*; when we are around others who are kind, it raises our energy. A famous quote by Wayne W. Dyer is very powerful: "When you have a choice to be right or to be kind, always pick kind."[27] The three aspects of kindness are kindness to ourselves, kindness to others, and others being kind to us. Each is discussed below.

Kristin Neff, PhD, is a leading expert in self-compassion and has written several books on the subject. Her research has shown that when we are kind to ourselves, we are less likely to be anxious, stressed, and depressed, and we are happier and more positive about our future. She states that there are many ways to practice self-compassion, such as journaling, positive self-talk, self-compassion meditation, and challenging our inner critic. She also gives tips on how to accomplish this by accepting the present moment, even if painful, and embracing ourselves with kindness, remembering that we are all imperfect humans.

For some people, their pain can increase initially as they learn how to open their heart to unconditionally love themselves. To experience self-compassion, you need to learn how—either with a psychologist or through guided meditations—that can be found for free on Dr. Neff's website self-compassion.org[28] and where she discusses seven key benefits of practicing *kindness to ourselves*:

1. **Self-soothing:** Using kind, supportive words to yourself can trigger the release of the chemical oxytocin, which increases feeling of trust, safety, and calmness.

2. **Better self-esteem:** When we give ourselves grace for our mistakes, we accept that a mistake is just a mistake, not a reflection of who we are.

3. **Higher life satisfaction:** "When we can view mistakes and setbacks as areas of growth and learning opportunities instead of as a negative reflection of our character, we often feel much better about our lives overall."

4. **More fulfilling relationships:** The more kindness we show ourselves, the easier it is to show kindness to others.

5. **Fewer symptoms of anxiety and depression:** When we are critical of ourselves, we activate the fight-or-flight response that can trigger anxiety and depression symptoms.

6. **Increased motivation to take risks:** When we take risks, there is always a possibility of failure, so when we show ourselves compassion, it's easier to accept the possible setbacks.

7. **Promotes a growth mindset:** Self-compassion allows you to have an open mind, giving you more confidence to explore and engage with anything that challenges your worldview.

The second aspect of kindness is *kindness to others*. Being kind to others not only helps others, but it also benefits us by increasing our connectivity with them, decreasing loneliness, combating low mood, reducing anxiety and depression, and improving relationships. This is such an important concept that November 13 is World Kindness Day. According to SSM Health, those who practice kindness have better health due to the biological changes that can occur while being kind to others, such as boosting levels of serotonin and dopamine and releasing oxytocin. In addition, kindness can lower blood pressure and the stress hormone cortisol, improving cardiac health.

As we all know, kindness is the act of being genuine about doing something to benefit someone else without considering our own needs. Ways to show kindness to others include volunteering, saying "thank you," being considerate, listening to someone, picking up trash, focusing on others, and so many other ways that they can't all be listed. Mentalhealth.org gives some tips to remember to show kindness: do something you enjoy such as sharing a skill with someone who has that interest and keeping others in mind by focusing on consideration. Don't overdo kindness by exerting too much energy, time, or money as it can cause stress. Volunteering in an area of interest increases feelings of self-esteem, social connection, and well-being. Or do something to benefit a cause you believe in.[29] While there are so many ways to show kindness to others, which benefits them and us, it is important to be around people who are kind to us, which is the third aspect of kindness.

Being around people who are kind to us is just as important as being kind to others. When people are mean to us, our mental health is negatively affected. Studies suggest that being around negative people may lead to depression, anxiety, and physical symptoms. No one wants to be around a bully because it makes us feel bad, but even being around rude people can have the same effect because our brain perceives it as a threat and leads to irritability and stress. Disrespectful people are also a problem because it may cause fear, anger, shame, self-doubt, depression, and many other negative feelings. The point here is to surround yourself with people who are kind and limit time with people who are mean, rude, or disrespectful. The next chapter has more details on the effects of being around positive and negative people.

Author and internationally renowned Japanese scientist Dr. Masaru Emoto photographed water crystals to demonstrate the effect that words have on water.[30] This is significant because our bodies are mostly water (60% for men and 55% for women) and it demonstrates how words effect our bodies.

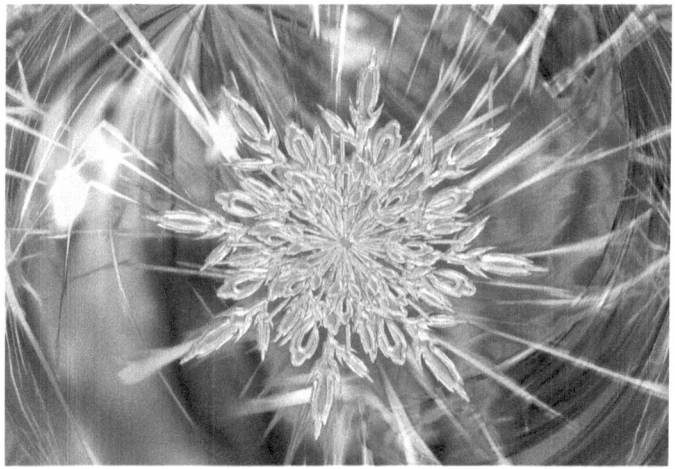

Sample of a water crystal exposed to positive emotions

Dr. Emoto spent 20 years taking samples of water under different circumstances, freezing the water, and observing it under a microscope to see crystals form. It is truly amazing to see how water crystals change depending on what they are exposed to. The crystals from contaminated water, exposed to heavy metal music and mean words, thoughts, or intentions were all ugly and nonsymmetrical; crystals from clean, fresh water, exposed to healing music, and kind words, thoughts, or intentions created beautiful symmetrical water crystals.

If this seems unbelievable, I suggest you try an experiment to see how powerful words are. A rice experiment, which I have done several times, proves the observations Dr. Emoto made are legitimate: Put two containers of cooked rice, which holds a lot of water, in separate locations. On one container, write something positive like *kindness*, and when walking by it, talk to the rice kindly. For example, you might say, "You are so beautiful. I love you." On the other container, write something negative, such as *meanness*, and when walking by it, talk to it in a mean way. You might say something like, "I hate you. You are disgusting." I was amazed to see what happened after several weeks; the rice that was spoken to in a mean manner turned moldy quickly, whereas the rice that was spoken to in a kind manner stayed white much longer. If you are interested, YouTube videos can teach you how to perform the experiment.

A final thought on kindness: kindness is contagious. When you are kind, that energy will come back to you. As discussed earlier, like attracts like—the law of attraction. So, the kinder you are to people and yourself, the more likely you will have kindness returned to you.

Suggestion: Surround yourself with kind people, use kind words to others, and practice self-compassion.

6

....

Positive People

*If you hang out with chickens, you are going to cluck,
and if you hang out with eagles, you're going to fly.*
—Dr. Steve Maraboli

For someone dealing with mental health issues, being around positive people is extremely important, as negative people can drain your energy and influence your thinking. An article in the *Times of India*[31] states that there are many benefits of being around positive people.

1. **They influence you:** By being around positive people, you begin to embrace their positive qualities.

2. **They help you better manage stress:** Associating with positive people helps you cope with life's stresses.

3. **It improves your physical health:** Psychologist Shilagh Mirgain says positive thinking can improve physical health.

4. **They help you make better choices:** Positive people can assist you in making realistic, beneficial, and positive decisions.

5. **They help you become successful:** Positive people will boost your confidence and strengthen your resilience, which can lead to more success.

6. **They keep you away from negativity.**

7. **They motivate you to follow your dreams and goals.**

While it is important to surround yourself with positive people, it is not always possible to avoid negative people, but you can protect yourself from their negative energy. For example, you can ignore the perpetrator, move to a different space, look away from the person, change the conversation into a positive one, or use imagery. *The National Library of Medicine*[32] reports studies that show a correlation between negative people and depression and anxiety, so it is important to be surrounded by positive people.

How do you know if someone has negative energy that you want to avoid? The Marque Medical Clinic says negativity can manifest in several ways.[33]

1. Cynicism

2. Hostility

3. Filtering: Only noticing the bad

4. Polarized thinking: If something is not perfect, it must be horrible

5. Jumping to conclusions

6. Catastrophizing

7. Blaming

8. Emotional reasoning: Using emotions to define what's real and what isn't

9. Fallacy of change: Thinking that If people or circumstances changed, they'd be happy

10. Heaven's reward fallacy: Assuming a reward, which doesn't come, and becoming depressed

When I was studying to become a practitioner in Science of Mind[34] several years ago, I created a list of positive behaviors we want to embrace and be around and negative behaviors to avoid. The idea is that we want to be around positive behaviors more to overcome the negative behaviors we might encounter. I'm sure there are other behaviors you can think of, but this is a start.

Positive	Negative
love	hate
peace	hostility
compassion	judgment
kindness	meanness
generosity	greed
gratitude	jealousy
forgiveness	fear
grace	ego
surrender	closed thinking
integrity	guilt
hopefulness	hopelessness
acceptance	denial
openheartedness	closed heartedness
rest	sleep deprivation
honesty	deception
joy	sadness
confidence	doubt
right thinking	wrong thinking
optimism	cynicism

Suggestion: Surround yourself with positive people and limit the amount of time you spend with negative people.

7

Positive Self-Affirmations

Every thought we think is creating our future.
—Louise Hay

Positive self-affirmations have many benefits, but what are they? Wellspring Center for Prevention[35] defines it as "a phrase or quote you say to yourself in order to combat or challenge overwhelming negative thoughts." Positive affirmations may be self-affirmations, goal-oriented affirmations, or healing affirmations. The following are some examples:

1. Today is a great day.

2. I can do it.

3. I am enough.

4. Everything is okay.

5. Today, I choose to be confident.

6. I am healthy.

7. I am kind.

8. I have everything I need.

Examples are endless, but one of the most powerful uses of self-affirmations is mirror work according to Louise L. Hay, author of *You Can Heal Your Life*.[36] When you say a positive self-affirmation to yourself in front of the mirror, the mirror reflects to you the feelings you have about yourself. This is important because the feelings reflected back to you inform you of beliefs that need to change. You can also write down your self-affirmations and tape them on something, like your mirror or refrigerator, to remind yourself of them. This will help you create a habit.

Scientific studies show the benefits of positive affirmations include increased feelings of self-worth and motivation, decreased stress levels, reduced negative thoughts, improved sleep, and a more positive mood. Wellspring Center for Prevention[37] lists some helpful tips:

1. **Be consistent:** Have a routine to practice daily.

2. **Involve loved ones:** If you have a hard time coming up with something positive to say to yourself, ask a friend or family member for help.

3. **Start slow:** Start with one affirmation a day, then increase as you become more comfortable.

4. **Combine your affirmations with an action:** For example, if your affirmation is "I am calm" and something upsets you, practice deep breathing.

5. **Create your own affirmations:** Base them on whatever you are struggling with the most.

6. **Set your affirmations in the present:** This helps you believe the statement is true *right now* (see below).

7. **Get personal and specific:** Base them on real, specific traits.

8. **Be patient with yourself:** Be kind to yourself, knowing that change can be slow.

As discussed in tip number six above, it is important to say your affirmations in the present tense. I've studied this extensively with my training in Science of Mind and have practiced it for probably 15 years.

A multitude of books on this subject are available, but here are the first books that taught me this principle:

The Secret by Rhonda Byrne[38]

Miracles by Stuart Wilde[39]

You'll See It When You Believe It by Wayne Dyer[40]

Super Attractor by Gabrielle Bernstein[41]

I Am Source Code by Dr. Janette Marie Freeman[42]

I know from experience that saying your affirmations in the present tense allows that energy to manifest. An example of how this has worked for me: I wrote several letters to myself to manifest things in my life. One of them was about growing my fingernails. While that might not seem important to someone else, it has bothered me my whole life. I was a nailbiter for as long as I can remember. As an adult, I decided to get acrylic nails to avoid biting them. It worked beautifully, but when the COVID-19 pandemic hit, nail salons closed. Because I could not continue getting acrylic nails, I started biting them again until I wrote a letter to myself in the present tense. I put this letter in a shoebox and forgot about it but then I noticed helpful things started showing up—my sister-in-law told me about a supplement called Bone Up that helped strengthen her nails, so I started using it. Another thing just popped in my head; I remembered that when I had my nails professionally done, the tech always put a cuticle softener on my nails so I started doing that because biting my cuticles would lead to biting my nails. Five years after the pandemic, I have quit biting my nails. I attribute this to the positive affirmation I wrote back in 2020.

Suggestion: Start a practice of daily self-affirmations. If you need help getting started, there are many examples of affirmations available online.

8

....

Forgiveness

Forgiveness is the greatest gift you can give yourself.
It's not for the other person.
—Maya Angelou

Forgiveness is hard for a lot of people because they think that if they forgive someone, they are denying or condoning the offense, but that is not true. While there are many different ways to look at forgiveness, a general definition according to the Greater Good Science Center is "a conscious decision to release feelings of resentment or vengeance toward a person or group who has harmed you, regardless of whether they actually deserve your forgiveness."[43] The other aspect of forgiveness is to forgive ourselves, which seems harder for many people than forgiving others. Let's discuss self-forgiveness first, since as discussed in the section on energy in chapter 25, a suicidal person who has feelings of self-loathing and lacks self-forgiveness just perpetuates this belief, whereas self-forgiveness is associated with lower levels of anxiety and depression.

Since any type of forgiveness is a deliberate act, verywellmind.com suggests seven steps to forgive yourself[44]:

1. **Understand your emotions:** Become aware of the emotions you are experiencing.

2. **Accept responsibility for your actions:** Accept your actions and show yourself compassion; this is the hardest step because you stop justifying your actions.

3. **Treat yourself with kindness and compassion:** Having self-compassion as you show remorse for your actions.

4. **Express remorse for your mistake:** It is normal to feel guilty as you express your remorse, and it can be beneficial as you move toward positive change.

5. **Make amends and apologize:** Look for ways to make it up to the person you hurt.

6. **Learn from the experience:** Use your mistake as a learning opportunity to make better choices in the future.

7. **Try to do better:** Remind yourself of the mistake you made and the guilt you experienced to guide your actions in the future.

In the article "Forgiveness: Letting Go of Grudges and Bitterness," the Mayo Clinic[45] states the many benefits forgiveness in general, such as healthier relationships, improved mental health, less anxiety, stress, and hostility, fewer symptoms of depression, and improved self-esteem. Holding a grudge and harboring feelings of resentment and bitterness is harmful to us. One of my favorite quotes by Marianne Williamson is "Unforgiveness is like drinking poison yourself and waiting for the other person to die." When we are unwilling to forgive others or ourselves, we are just hurting ourselves. If you are having trouble holding a grudge or forgiving someone who hurt you, especially if they don't take responsibility for their actions, the article lists a few things you can try.

1. Practice empathy; try to see the situation from their point of view

2. Ask yourself what circumstances could have caused the person to behave as they did

3. Reflect on times you have been forgiven

4. Write in a journal

5. Pray

6. Use a guided meditation

7. Realize that forgiveness is a process

Another option is regular sessions with a counselor who can offer you more strategies. YouTube also has videos that can be helpful.

> **Suggestion:** Practice forgiving yourself and others on a regular basis using the suggestions above.

9

Pharmaceuticals

About a third of Americans are taking a prescription medication
that could potentially cause depression or increase suicide risk.
—JAMA[46]

Writing about prescription medications is tricky because I have a biased opinion due to the situation with my son. From my research, I have discovered that there are over 200 medications that cause suicidal side effects—not just antidepressants.[47] Research on vox.com[48] shows suicidal side effects from some anticonvulsants, analgesics, anxiolytics, hypnotics, and sedatives, gastrointestinal agents, hormones/hormone modifiers, respirator agents, antihypertensives, corticosteroids, birth control pills, beta blockers, proton pump inhibitors, and others. To be listed on a prescription, 1% to 2% of patients must have experienced the side effects. Therefore, each person must work with their primary care physician and/or psychiatrist to carefully consider the potential side effects of any medication.

Many medications prescribed for mental health issues temporarily improve the symptoms but do not address the cause. Pharmaceuticals are often prescribed by a psychiatrist—who has completed medical school and has acquired knowledge on medications—after making a diagnosis using the *Diagnostic and Statistical Manual of Mental Disorders* (DSM). Controversies surround the use of the DSM because of overdiagnosis or stigmatizing individuals with mental health issues.

Brain imaging scans, such as SPECT imaging described in Chapter 3, can show which part of the brain is affected. According to the Amen Clinics,[49] this takes the guesswork out of diagnosis; along with a full evaluation, this scan is reviewed by a physician who makes personalized recommendations that can include medications, supplements, psychotherapy, and so on.

Psychotherapy along with pharmaceuticals has been proven to work best for people suffering from mild to moderate depression. It is important to note differences between psychiatrist and psychologist treatments, beginning with their training. While both approaches use talk therapy, psychiatrists are trained to deal with diagnosis, prevention, and treatment of mental health conditions. Their treatments involve psychosocial interventions, medication, and interventional treatments including electroconvulsive therapy (ECT), and transcranial magnetic stimulation (TMS). Psychologist training can include a variety of therapies including cognitive behavior therapy (CBT), dialectical behavior therapy (DBT), exposure therapy (ET), interpersonal therapy (IT), eye movement depensation and reprocessing therapy (EMDR), mentalization-based therapy (MBT), pet therapy (PT), and psychodynamic therapy (PT).

The National Library of Medicine states three types of antidepressants usually prescribed to treat the most common form of depression—unipolar depression: tricyclic antidepressants (TCAs), selective serotonin reuptake inhibitors (SSRIs), and selective serotonin noradrenaline reuptake inhibitors (SNRIs).[50] These drugs can be effective for moderate, severe, and chronic depression but do not help everyone. Studies have shown that antidepressants improved symptoms in only about 20% more people than those in a placebo group.

SSRI and SNRI medications adjust the brain's levels of *serotonin*—a neurotransmitter that acts like a hormone and carries signals between neurons—and blocks the reabsorption (reuptake) of serotonin into neurons, making more serotonin available to improve the transmission of messages between neurons. Natural ways to increase serotonin in the brain include tryptophan-containing foods, sunlight, certain supplements, and exercising regularly. Amitriptyline is used to treat depression by increasing endorphins in the brain. But again, natural ways to increase endorphins in the brain are discussed in this book and include exercise, acupuncture, meditation, sex, music, laughter, and ultraviolet light.

When medications don't help with depression, treatment-resistant depression (TRD) is likely the issue (see Chapter 2). Jennifer Coughlin, MD (co-founder and co-director of Johns Hopkins' Brain Health Program) and Ana Soule, CRNP (psychiatric nurse practitioner at the Brain Health Program)[51] state that 30% of people diagnosed with major depressive disorder have TRD, meaning there was no improvement after trying multiple drugs. They recommend next steps such as a second opinion from a specialist in depression, psychoeducation to learn about the length of time needed to see benefits from the medication, and exploring other risk factors for depression with a psychiatrist.

Suggestion: Discuss the options with a reputable psychologist and psychiatrist, then research each one to determine which treatment is the safest and most effective.

10

Social Media

There is a valid reason social media is linked to depression and loneliness . . . people spend countless hours a day online strolling through the timeline of others with envy, regret, and little appreciation for their own life.
—Germany Kent

While there can be some positive aspects to social media use, research says the negative outweighs the positives. Vantage Fit, a global employee wellness platform, examined how social media affects mental health.[52]The main reason why social media is harmful to mental health is because people compare themselves to others and this leads to feelings of anxiety, depression, and loneliness. The following is a list of the negative aspects of social media use listed on their blog:

1. Decreased attention span

2. Detachment from the real world

3. Developing feelings of envy, jealousy, and loneliness

4. Excessive fear of losing out or anxiety

5. Triggers feelings of inadequacy

6. Increases risk of depression

7. Builds addiction

8. Increases risk of self-harm and suicidal thoughts

9. Increases feelings of self-absorption

10. Disrupts healthy sleep patterns

The US Surgeon General's Advisory on social media and youth mental health[53] discusses the negative impact of social media on children and adolescents. Not everyone using social media is affected in the same way because of many factors—such as individual strengths and vulnerabilities, cultural, historical, and socioeconomic factors—but ages 10–19 is a critical time for adolescents' brain development; the brain is more susceptible to risk-taking behaviors and depression usually emerges during this time.

The report also states that about 64% of youth are exposed to hate-based content and some social media platforms show content that has been linked to childhood deaths, such as self-harm-related content and suicide. It was also found that excessive social media use was related to poor sleep quality.

Another problem with social media is that adolescents spend too much time on it ; in 2023, a Gallup survey by Jonathan Rothwell said 51% of adolescents spend 4.8 hours per day on social media—mostly on YouTube and TikTok.[54] Fortunately, many platforms have been listening to parents' concerns and now include controls so parents can limit the time and/or content their children can access. Many studies demonstrate the dangers of excessive social media usage, but the point is to limit the usage and control the content your child can access.

Suggestion: Limit social media to 30 minutes a day and use parental controls to limit the content that can be viewed.

11

....

Watching News and Television

*TV does not care about you or what happens to you. It's downright
bad for your mental health now, and that's not a far-out concept . . .
It is bad for your physical health and your mental health.*
—Tom Petty

We've all heard that watching too much TV is not good for our health,
but did you know it can cause increased anxiety and depression?
Binge-watching is particularly problematic; studies show the correlation between binge-watching and anxiety, depression, insomnia, and
loneliness. Engaging in mentally passive activities, such as watching
TV, can increase the risk of depression by 43%. A recommendation is
to replace some of the TV time with brain-stimulating activities such
as puzzles and reading.[55]

An article written by Maureen Salamon at Harvard Medical School
states that four or more hours of TV a day increases the risk of several
illnesses including depression, and that there is a 35% greater risk of
depression when watching four hours of TV compared to less than
two hours.[56] One of the most detrimental aspects of watching TV is
watching the news.

Johns Hopkins University and Medicine published the article
"Protecting Our Mental Health from Negative News Coverage."[57] News
coverage is available 24 hours a day and watching it can increase anxiety and depression. One study showed that watching only 14 minutes

of news had this effect; the news is often sensationalized and shows upsetting footage, triggering our fight-or-flight response to release adrenaline and cortisol. Additionally, be mindful of the sources of news you view as there is a lot of fake news. Another problem is that over 50% of people get their news from social media that uses algorithms to keep them coming back for more.

To offset this problem, determine what triggers anxiety and depression for you then limit your consumption of those subjects. You might also read the news instead of watching it as there will be less disturbing imagery. While the article recommended watching no more than 30 minutes of news daily, even 14 minutes can trigger anxiety and depression, so limit your time watching news and get involved in things you are passionate about and 1. give you a sense of purpose. Additionally, be mindful of the sources of news as there is a lot of fake news out there.

> **Suggestion:** Watch less than two hours of TV daily, limit news consumption to no more than 14 minutes a day and replace TV time with brain-stimulating activities; check Google for brain-stimulating activities and ideas.

12

Drugs and Alcohol

*Remember, just because you hit bottom
doesn't mean you have to stay there.*
—Robert Downey Jr.

The use of drugs and/or alcohol is problematic for anyone struggling with anxiety or depression. Reasons for someone to use these substances include genetics, the desire to self-medicate, and existing mental illness. The main idea of this very complex issue is that drugs and alcohol negatively affect the function of the brain, so it is best to avoid them. That is easier said than done, but specialized programs can help people to quit using these substances.

From my research, I've found that abusing drugs can result in mental health illnesses such as schizophrenia, bipolar disorder, manic depression, ADHD, generalized anxiety disorder, obsessive-compulsive disorder, PTSD, panic disorder, and antisocial personality. The most common illnesses resulting from alcohol abuse are depressive disorders, anxiety disorders, trauma- and stress-related disorders, and sleep disorders.

However, a person may be using these substances to self-medicate because they already have a mental illness. Whatever the reason for the abuse, it is best to stop using drugs and alcohol. Addiction, referred to as substance use disorder (SUD), is mainly due to brain dysfunction according to the Amen Clinic (SPECT imaging can pinpoint the area of the brain affected).[58] The clinic's website states that treatment needs to be individualized since there are six types of addicts. Some other treatment options:

1. Alcoholics Anonymous and Narcotics Anonymous 12-step program[59]

2. American Addiction Centers[60]

3. The Salvation Army USA[61]

4. RehabPath[62]

5. FindTreatment.gov[63]

6. SAMHSA: Substance Abuse and Mental Health Services Administration[64]

More resources can be found online, and some treatment programs may be only local, but regardless of where the help comes from, it is important to stop abusing drugs and/or alcohol as it does more harm than good.

Suggestion: Do not use drugs or alcohol; if they are already being abused, speak to a health care provider for guidance on choosing a treatment plan.

~ V ~

Introduction: Body

Taking care of your physical body is good for your mental health.
—Unknown

This section of the book focuses on ways to take care of your physical body. The mind and body are interconnected, so when you take care of your body, you are taking care of your mental health. Proper nutrition is one of the most beneficial things you can do for yourself. This section discusses how the lack of nutrients is linked to depression and anxiety, along with supplements that can be helpful. Traditional Chinese Medicine and the herbs used in it gives another approach to dealing with physical problems.

Everyday practices are beneficial to our mental health as well, such as sleep, hydration, exercise, movement, and grounding discussed in this section. Finally, I outline the benefits of massage, chiropractic therapy, acupuncture, acupressure, and emotional freedom technique.

Suggestion: Focus on the daily practices of adequate sleep, enough water, and exercise first. Then learn about nutrition and make necessary changes to diet. Follow up with any of the other practices that resonate with you.

13

....

Nutrition

Let food be thy medicine and medicine be thy food.
—Hippocrates (400 BC)

Many people do not consider nutrition when looking to help someone with mental health issues, but nutrition plays a key role in how our brain functions. This makes sense because depression starts in the brain, as do all our functions. Inflammation causes many health-related illnesses such as cancer but can also cause mental health problems. Studies show the correlation between mental health issues and mineral deficiencies. In *Nutrition and Mental Health*, Dr. David Thomas summarized the findings of 214 peer-reviewed papers published from 1940 to 2002.[65] Conditions associated with mineral deficiencies included ADHD, anxiety, aggression, bipolar disorder, depression, PMS, and schizophrenia.

Our bodies need macronutrients and micronutrients to function properly; a diet low in nutrients causes inflammation in the brain. When the recommended daily/dietary allowance (RDA) was established in 1941 by the United States National Research Council, the brain was not a consideration. Therefore, the recommendations we have now are not high enough for individuals who have mental health issues. There are several reasons for this, but the main idea is that individuals with a mental illness may need a higher level of micronutrients that the RDA has established.

Proper nutrition is one way to activate the neurotransmitters that affect mood.

Neurotransmitters are chemical messengers that help nerve cells communicate with each other. They include serotonin, dopamine, glutamate, and acetylcholine. Neurotransmitters serve several functions, such as regulation of appetite, the sleep-wake cycle, and mood. Low levels of neurotransmitters can lead to problems.

—*Verywell Health*[66]

In *The Better Brain: Overcome Anxiety, Combat Depression, and Reduce ADHD and Stress with Nutrition*, the authors cite much research that supports this.[67] Although many studies show the benefits of individual vitamins and minerals, the authors believe that the body needs higher levels of all of them. In addition to vitamins and minerals, the body needs the correct ratio of omega 3 to omega 6 fatty acids.

Omega 3 fatty acids include alpha-linolenic acid (ALA) found in walnuts, chia seeds, and flaxseeds. Marine-based omega 3 fatty acids are eicosatetraenoic acid (EPA) and docosahexaenoic (DHA) found mostly in seafood. These acids are critical for brain function but since they are not vegan, it is difficult to get enough DHA and EPA if a person does not eat seafood. A couple of other options include algae oil, seaweed, nori, spirulina, and chlorella. One of the best ways to get more omega 3 fatty acids is to eat whole, unprocessed foods. Studies have shown that the optimal eating pattern is the Mediterranean diet that includes lettuce, apples, berries, carrots, leafy vegetables, cucumbers, citrus fruits, lean fish, and seeds. Whole foods are best for our bodies, but we still might not be getting enough nutrition due to factors such as depletion of minerals in the soil and the effects of using pesticides.

Many American diets are too high in processed foods and the ratio of omega 6 fatty acids (polyunsaturated fatty acids) to omega 3 fatty acids is too high. Also, foods high in omega 6 fatty acids lack essential vitamins and minerals our bodies need. The omega 6 fatty acids to omega 3 fatty acids ratio should be 1:1 or 2:1, but ultra-processed foods have a ratio of about 20:1. This is a problem because elevated levels of omega 6 fatty acids may contribute to inflammation.

Processed foods high in omega 6 fatty acids include crackers and chips, fast food, soybean oil, corn oil, mayonnaise, sunflower seeds, almonds, walnuts, and cashews. Foods high in omega 3 fatty acids are mackerel, salmon, cod liver oil, herring, oysters, sardines, anchovies, caviar, flaxseeds, chia seeds, walnuts, and soybeans.

Clearly, a nutritious diet plays a key role in optimal mental health. While it is not always possible to get adequate nutrition from the foods we eat, supplements can be added to a healthy diet. Authors of the book *The Better Brain* discuss several supplements that have been shown to have mental health benefits, such as EMPowerplus Advanced (EMP)[68] and Daily Essential Nutrients (DEN).[69] The authors say the supplements should be tried for at least three months to determine whether they are helpful, but when transitioning from medication, six months to a year may be required (with a physician's input).

> **Suggestion:** Consider a Mediterranean diet and include foods rich in the omega 3 fatty acids, DHA, and EPA. Also, consider a nutritional supplement by researching the two listed above.

14

....

Supplements

*Getting all the nutrients you need
simply cannot be done without supplements.*
—Steven Gundry

A nutritious diet is important for brain function, but it is not always possible to get adequate nutrition from the foods we eat. Several supplements have proved to be helpful for depression according to Daniel K. Hall-Flavin, MD, at the Mayo Clinic.[70] Below is a list of several supplements, but remember they are not replacements for a healthy diet, medical diagnosis, or treatment. It is important to note that some supplements interfere with certain medications and should not be started without discussing with your doctor.

1. **St. John's wort:** This supplement is not approved by the FDA but may help mild to moderate depression. Be cautious if taking other medications; it can interfere with their efficacy. **Do not use** if on antidepressants; it can cause serious side effects.

2. **SAMe (s-adenosylmethionine):** Not approved by the FDA for treating depression; more research is needed to determine its effectiveness. **Do not use** while on antidepressants; it may have serious side effects or trigger mania in some with bipolar disorder.

3. **Omega 3 fatty acids:** These fatty acids are found in marine sources such as fish, algae oil, etc. While more research is needed, they are generally safe but may leave a fishy aftertaste.

4. **Saffron:** More studies are needed but saffron oil may improve symptoms of depression; however, high doses can cause significant side effects.

5. **5-HTP (5-hydroxytryptophan):** This supplement may play a role in increasing serotonin level, but more research is needed; **do not take** with certain antidepressants; it can have serious side effects.

6. **DHEA (dehydroepiandrosterone):** This is a hormone our bodies make. Preliminary studies have shown depression symptoms improve when taking DHEA; it is usually well tolerated but has the potential for serious side effects if taken in large doses or long-term.

Supplements have been found to help reduce anxiety too. People suffering from anxiety are often prescribed a selective serotonin reuptake inhibitor (SSRI) and many supplements can work in the same way. Dr. Leslie Madrak, a board-certified integrative medicine and addiction medicine psychiatrist with Jefferson Health says these supplements can work for anxiety. "They can help the body reabsorb neurotransmitters, like serotonin, to help reduce anxiety the same way a medication like Prozac would."[71] Again, dangerous interactions with some prescriptions are possible; never start supplements without discussing it with your doctor first. Below are the supplements recommended by Dr. Madrak.

1. **Vitamin D3:** A deficiency can hinder mental well-being; 15-20 minutes of sunlight a day is recommended, but it's not always possible, especially in the winter months. Suggested daily dose: 2,000 international units (IU), but if there is a deficiency, a larger dosage might be needed.

2. **Magnesium:** Magnesium is also helpful for insomnia. Suggested daily dose: Up to 200 milligrams (mg) before bed.

3. **Melatonin:** Commonly used for insomnia, it is safe to take with prescriptions since it's a naturally occurring hormone in our bodies. Suggested daily dose: 1.0 mg to 10 mg before bed.

4. **Omega 3 fatty acids:** Found in fish oil, krill oil, flaxseeds, chia seeds, spinach, and Brussel sprouts. Suggested daily dose: 1,000 mg to 2,000 mg.

5. **Chamomile:** Often found in tea. Be cautious of overconsumption if taking blood thinners. Suggested daily dose: 800 mg to 1,600 mg about 30 minutes before bed.

6. **Valerian root:** Be cautious if taking a sedating medication as well. Suggested daily dose: 300 mg to 600 mg before bed.

7. **Ashwagandha:** Highly recommended because it decreases cortisol (stress hormone) levels. Suggested daily dose: 500 mg to 1,000 mg.

8. **Kava:** This controversial supplement has been known to have "euphoric" effects. Be cautious if you take sedative medication. Suggested daily dose: 1,000 mg to 1,400 mg.

One more supplement to consider for anxiety is gamma-aminobutyric acid (GABA). After my son died, I had severe anxiety and started taking GABA twice a day. After a few months, I was able to stop taking antianxiety medications altogether. There are not many side effects, but it can lower blood pressure and should not be taken if pregnant or breastfeeding. Again, always talk to your doctor first.

A final supplement available is a trace mineral supplement. Because a person with mental illness may need more minerals than are recommended by the RDA, this is an easy way to add the minerals into the diet, either through liquid drops or capsules. An abstract on the National Institute of Health website discusses mineral deficiencies and other dietary problems associated with depression.[72] Studies have found that excessive sugar intake, diets low in protein, and obesity are associated with depression.

Suggestion: Before taking any supplements, meet with your doctor for blood tests and to discuss your options.

15

....

Sleep

The best bridge between despair and hope is a good night's sleep.
—E. Joseph Cossman

Quality sleep is critical for someone dealing with anxiety and depression, and there is a close link between depression and insomnia. Johns Hopkins Medicine states that 75% of depressed people have trouble either falling asleep or staying asleep.[73] This correlation could be due to depression or depression could be due to lack of sleep. Either way, getting a good night's sleep is important to maintaining good mental health.

Sleep requirements vary with age but here is a general guide.

Ages 3–5:   10–13 hours
Ages 6–12:   9–12 hours
Ages 13–18:   8–10 hours
Ages 18+:   7 hours

While the number of hours of sleep is important, the quality of sleep is just as important. Quality sleep involves falling asleep easily (within 30 minutes), staying asleep, and waking feeling refreshed. Harvard Health Publishing lists eight secrets to a good night's sleep.[74]

1. **Exercise in the morning:** "Exercise boosts the effect of natural sleep hormones such as melatonin."

2. **Reserve the bed for sleep and sex:** Avoid watching TV or using any electronics in bed.

3. **Keep it comfortable:** A quiet, dark, cool environment is ideal.

4. **Start a sleep ritual:** Examples include drinking warm milk or chamomile tea, taking a warm bath, or listening to calming music.

5. **Eat—but not too much:** It is best not to be hungry or full at bedtime; stop eating two to three hours before bed.

6. **Avoid alcohol and caffeine:** Caffeine is a stimulant and can keep you awake. Alcohol will make you sleepy but then can keep you awake during the night. Also, avoid anything that will give you heartburn, such as citrus fruits/juices and spicy foods.

7. **De-stress:** Stress disrupts sleep because it activates fight-or-flight hormones. Meditation and deep breathing are beneficial.

8. **Get checked:** See your doctor if you have restless leg syndrome (discussed next), sleep apnea, or gastroesophageal reflux disease (GERD).

Sugary foods before bed also contribute to poor sleep quality and the ability to fall asleep quickly. Don't eat sweets for two to three hours before bedtime to avoid blood sugar and insulin spikes. Many studies have shown the correlation between sugary, ultra-processed foods and poor sleep. Some foods and drinks such as coffee, soda, and chocolate also have caffeine. It's generally recommended to stop caffeine intake six hours before bed.

Restless leg syndrome (RLS) occurs in 8% of Americans and is another contributing factor to poor sleep. RLS is considered a neurological disorder as well as a sleep disorder. It is characterized by the urge to get up due to a variety of uncomfortable symptoms such as legs that are achy, itchy, throbbing, have a pulling sensation or a crawling sensation, a feeling of electric shocks or needles. In a video called "Get Your ZZZs," a neurologist and speech specialist at Weill Cornell Medicine, Dr. Daniel Barone, describes the URGE criteria for diagnosing RLS as: U = the urge to move legs, R = symptoms occur at rest, G = get up and symptoms go away, E = evening is when symptoms occur.[75]

Idiopathic RLS, the most common type, is genetic or has an undetermined cause. Secondary RLS is triggered by something else, like a menstruating woman becoming low in iron due to blood loss or taking antihistamines at night. Treatment for RLS is treating the underlying cause if it can be determined; if a person is low in iron, iron supplements can be taken. If the cause is unknown, a doctor can prescribe dopamine or gabapentin medications to help alleviate the symptoms.

Naps are another consideration for getting enough sleep. The Mayo Clinic lists the pros and cons of napping.[76]

Napping benefits	Napping drawbacks
relaxation	feeling groggy right after waking
feeling less tired	trouble sleeping at night
more alert	
improved mental performance	
better mood	

Short (20–30 minute) naps before 3 p.m. are the most beneficial because you are less likely to wake up groggy and your nighttime sleep won't be disrupted. Experts warn that napping too long can disrupt your nighttime sleep so be sure to set an alarm to avoid this.

While a doctor may prescribe a sleep medication, it is best to try the eight secrets above first. Also, high-quality sheets, pillows, and mattresses help. Another consideration is to ensure beauty products used (night cream, hair growth serums, etc.) do not contain caffeine. Supplements helpful for a good night's sleep are valerian, magnesium, cannabidiol (CBD), cannabinol (CBN), melatonin, German chamomile, and passionflower. Lavendar oil and crystals next to the bed can be used, especially amethyst, selenite, lepidolite, or clear quartz because they have calming and sleep-enhancing properties. More information on the benefits of crystals is found in Chapter 31.

Suggestion: Strive for the recommended hours of sleep by using the eight sleep secrets and any other natural remedy listed above. Always discuss supplements with your doctor as they may have side effects when taken with certain medications.

16

....

Water

Increasing your water intake will promote happiness,
allowing your brain to continue making serotonin.
—www.cnet.com

The human body is made of primarily water, so it is important to consume enough water every day. Even though the body is made of around 60% water, the brain is 75% to 80% water; water in the brain is necessary for the production of hormones and neurotransmitters. Water in the brain gives it energy to function.

Benefits of drinking enough water include staying hydrated, improving digestion, weight management, cognitive clarity, muscle function, and flushing out toxins. While I could list many more benefits, there are also consequences when enough water is not consumed: include a lack of concentration, memory difficulties, and most importantly, your brain won't get enough tryptophan to convert to serotonin (the happy chemical). Dehydration depletes the levels of other amino acids in the brain. This can lead to feelings of anxiety and irritability.

New research links depression to dehydration.[77] Because dehydration causes the brain to function improperly, it is more difficult to fight depression. Dehydration also increases stress in the body—problematic because stress is a contributing factor to depression. Stress causes the adrenal glands to produce too much cortisol, stress hormone. CNET recommends women drink 11.5 cups of water per day; men should drink 15.5 cups per day.[78] An easy way to calculate how much water you should drink is to take your weight in pounds and drink half that amount in ounces according to Jennifer Stone,[79] PT, DPT, OCS, clinic supervisor at the University of Missouri System; if you weigh 150 pounds, aim to drink 75 ounces of water a day.

The quality of water you drink is also important. Alkaline water has a pH level of 6.5 to 8.5. Imbalanced pH levels can lead to physical and emotional issues. Frizzlife[80] states that drinking alkaline water instead of tap water helps balance the pH levels in the body and this can help reduce anxiety.

While drinking plenty of water is not a cure for anxiety or depression, it does help the brain function properly and combat symptoms. To get enough water each day, drink a glass of water in the morning, listen to your body if you feel thirsty, or set an alarm on your phone to remind you to drink water.

The Mayo Clinic also has recommendations to increase water intake.[81]

1. Flavor it by adding a slice of lemon or cucumber (or a flavor packet).

2. Tie it to a routine such as brushing your teeth or eating a meal.

3. Eat it through fruits and vegetables that have a high-water content.

4. Track it by marking a water bottle or tracking it on your smartphone.

5. Challenge a friend to see who can meet their goal the most often.

6. Take it on the go with a travel bottle.

7. Alternate your drinks if you enjoy soda or juice.

Increasing water consumption can be done, it just takes a little effort and planning.

> **Suggestion:** Incorporate some of the tips listed to drink enough water each day, e.g., halve your weight in pounds and drink that many ounces per day.

17

Grounding

*The moment one gives close attention to anything,
even a blade of grass, it becomes a mysterious, awesome,
indescribably magnificent world in itself.*
—Henry Miller

Grounding is a technique to connect you to the electrical charge of the earth that transfers electrons to your body. Benefits of grounding include easing stress, decreasing inflammation, and improving sleep. It also increases the levels of the feel-good chemical serotonin in the brain. You can ground yourself by being outside, barefoot on the earth walking or running, standing, sitting, or lying down on the earth.

You can also purchase a conductive pillow, grounding mat, or patches for grounding when sleeping. Using these may reduce nighttime levels of cortisol and can put you more in alignment with the natural 24-hour circadian rhythm. Note that there are possible side effects, such as flu-like symptoms, so it is best to discuss conductive material with your doctor first.

Grounding can be beneficial for someone with anxiety or depression; some studies have shown that one hour of grounding can significantly improve mood. Healthline.com offers 30 additional exercises for grounding to refocus on the present moment and distract you from anxious feelings.[82]

Physical grounding techniques:
1. Put your hand in cold water.
2. Pick up or touch items near you.
3. Breathe deeply.
4. Savor a food or drink.
5. Take a short walk.
6. Hold a piece of ice.
7. Savor a scent.
8. Move your body.
9. Listen to your surroundings.
10. Mentally feel your body.
11. Try the 5-4-3-2-1 method (described below).

Mental grounding techniques:
1. Play a memory game.
2. Think in categories.
3. Use math and numbers.
4. Recite something.
5. Make yourself laugh.
6. Use an anchoring statement.
7. Visualize a daily task you enjoy or don't mind doing.
8. Describe a common task.
9. Imagine yourself leaving painful feelings behind.
10. Describe what's around you.

Soothing grounding techniques:

1. Picture the voice or face of someone you love.

2. Practice self-kindness.

3. Sit with your pet.

4. List favorites.

5. Visualize your favorite place.

6. Plan an activity.

7. Touch something comforting.

8. List positive things.

9. Listen to music.

While there is not a lot of research explaining how grounding works, it is a common strategy for managing PTSD and anxiety. Grounding techniques help you stay in the present moment by focusing on your senses; what you can see, feel, hear, touch, and smell. To incorporate grounding, it might be helpful to practice these techniques when you are not feeling anxious so that you are comfortable using them. Also, when you are focusing on your environment, just describe it without thinking how you feel about it. It is a good idea to check in with yourself by recognizing your level of distress (1–10) before and after a grounding exercise to determine which technique is most useful.

5-4-3-2-1 Method: With this technique, you count backward from five to one and notice, for example, five things you see, four things you hear, three things you smell, two things you touch, and one thing you taste. Focusing on your senses encourages you to be fully present and aware of your surroundings, thus interrupting the anxiety. This method works by calming the nervous system. Videos online to help you learn this technique. *The Earthing Movie*, a documentary, might be helpful to understand grounding.

Suggestion: Try several different grounding techniques to find the ones that resonate with you and incorporate one of two into your daily routine.

18

....

Exercise and Movement

Exercise is the most potent and underrated antidepressant.
—Bill Phillips

I can't stress the importance of exercise enough because during exercise, the body releases endorphins, another mood boosting chemical, in the brain. Aerobic workouts, strength training, and yoga are some of the best exercises for this. According to the Mayo Clinic, "Research on depression, anxiety, and exercise shows that mental health and physical benefits also help mood and lessen anxiety."[83] Other benefits of regular exercise include reduced tension, stress, anger or frustration, and mental fatigue. It also gives us a natural energy boost, a sense of achievement, more focus and motivation, a healthier appetite, and fun.

The United States Department of Health and Human Services recommends 150 minutes of moderate aerobic activity a week or 75 minutes of vigorous aerobic activity per week.[84] This can be broken up throughout the day, but it is important to have daily physical activity of some sort. To get started, find a form of exercise that is enjoyable, discuss it with your primary care physician or psychologist for support, and set reasonable goals.

Some forms of exercise that might be enjoyable include jumping on a trampoline, walking, dancing, cycling, Tai Chi, Chi Quong, Chi Kung, martial arts, swimming, soccer, hiking, skateboarding, rollerblading, jumping rope, or gardening. Just be sure to choose something you like and follow through.

Suggestion: Choose an enjoyable activity and make it a goal to be active 20–30 minutes daily.

19

Yoga

*The meaning of yoga is connection of mind, body, and spirit. If you have
a bad telecommunication system, your body gets sick. Yoga helps fix that.*
—Bikram Choudhury

Yoga is an ancient Indian philosophy begun over 5,000 years ago. It
was used to promote spiritual growth and understanding in Hinduism,
Buddhism, and Jainism. The main purpose of yoga is to bring body
and mind together through movement, breathing, and meditation.
Today, yoga is practiced by many.

According to Aura Wellness Center, yoga can contribute to healing,
but it is not a magical cure for all ailments. Yoga creates "an awareness
that allows us to observe ourselves without judgment."[85] This helps us
understand our physical, emotional, and mental states. Practicing yoga
can help a person not only achieve physical fitness, such as increased
flexibility, strength, and balance, but also inner clarity, spiritual growth,
and transcendence. Additionally, it reduces stress levels, improves
sleep, reduces joint pain, and enhances cognitive function. Harvard
Medical School states that all exercise can improve mood by lowering
stress hormones and elevating endorphins (the feel-good chemical),
but yoga may also elevate levels of gamma-aminobutyric acid (GABA)
that is helpful for elevating mood and decreasing anxiety.[86]

Like all other practices discussed in this book, it should be used
in conjunction with other treatments under a doctor's care. A person

should see their physician before starting any new physical activity, especially if they have not been physically active for a while. To get started, check out YouTube videos online or local yoga studios for in-person classes.

Suggestion: Start out easy with a 10- to 15-minute YouTube video once or twice per week to learn some yoga basics. Increase gradually; if possible, take a yoga class in person.

20

....

Massage Therapy

*Regular massage therapy can boost your mood
and reduce stress hormones.*
—Glossgenious.com

Massage therapy has a multitude of benefits for our bodies, including reducing stress, anxiety, and depression. This practice has been around for over 5,000 years in many cultures throughout the world. The purpose of massage is generally for the treatment of body stress or pain. The Mayo Clinic's website[87] states that a therapist uses various levels of pressure on soft tissue, which includes muscles, connective tissue, tendons, ligaments, and skin. Massage therapy, a part of integrative medicine, helps relieve stress, lesson pain and muscle tightness, increase relaxation, and improve the work of the immune system.

National University of Health Sciences, a leader in the field of integrative medicine, gives four mental health benefits of regular massage.[88]

1. **Improves your relaxation skills:** Heart rate, blood pressure, oxygen consumption, and salivary cortisol levels decrease when you are relaxed; therefore, it reduces stress and anxiety.

2. **More efficient rest:** It improves the quality of your sleep.

3. **Alleviates the symptoms of chronic illnesses and diseases:** People with chronic illnesses and diseases have higher levels of stress.

4. **Increases your overall happiness:** Serotonin and dopamine (the feel-good chemicals) increase in the brain.

Types of massage to choose from include *Swedish* (percussion, kneading, vibration, tapping, and rolling), *chair* (focuses on neck, shoulders, and back), *deep tissue* (focuses on deeper layers of muscle and fascia), *Shiatsu* (applies pressure to points of your body as in acupuncture), *reflexology* (pressure on specific areas on your feet that correspond with other systems and organs in the body), *aromatherapy* (massage combined with essential oils), *cupping* (suction from cups stimulate the release of endorphins, which are the feel-good hormones), and *hot stone* (applies warm, flat stones to relax the muscles).

There are more types of massage, but this brief introduction gives you a place to start; look for a massage therapist in your area who practices the type of massage that interests you.

Suggestion: Choose a massage style you feel would benefit you and get two massages a week. If it is too expensive, start with a chair massage; you can find 15-minute sessions that are less costly.

Chiropractic Therapy

*The natural healing force within each of us
is the greatest force in getting well.*
—Hippocrates

You probably already know that chiropractic therapy focuses on alignment of the spine, but most people are not familiar with neurological-based chiropractic therapy—a holistic approach to improve physical symptoms and mental health. We need balance in our lives to function optimally, which includes spinal alignment, proper nutrition, exercise, and so on.

Benefits of neurological-based chiropractic therapy on our mental health according to an orthopedic clinic[89] are:

1. **Releases positive hormones:** Chiropractic adjustments release the hormones oxytocin and cortisol that can reduce stress and inflammation to improve overall mental health.

2. **Promotes sleep:** Studies have shown that chiropractic care can improve sleep patterns.

3. **Is an all-natural solution without side effects:** As opposed to medications that do have side effects.

4. **Lowers blood pressure:** High blood pressure can lead to anxiety and depression; lowering blood pressure decreases them.

5. **Relieves tension:** Anxiety and depression often cause muscle tension; chiropractic care works on musculoskeletal health to relieve muscle tightness and tension.

Find the right chiropractor, someone who is looking to give long-term results, not just a quick fix that doesn't last. With neurological-based chiropractic care, you can benefit long-term and stay healthy throughout your life. Three main reasons to pursue a neurologically based chiropractor according to Anchor Health[90] include the following.

1. **They correct underlying issues:** These chiropractors identify the deepest, most basic element that has caused the current situation.

2. **They provide immediate relief:** Patients can have short-term relief of symptoms, but the focus is on repeated sessions to work toward long-term relief.

3. **They** look to the future.

Another treatment a neurological-based chiropractor might offer is neurofeedback. While it has been used since the 1950s, neurofeedback has only been used in chiropractic therapy recently to treat anxiety, depression, and PTSD. Currently, only about 200 offices in the United States have integrated this therapy into their practice. Neurofeedback is a type of biofeedback that has to do with brain waves:

Neurofeedback is a method that assists subjects to control their brain waves consciously . . . the electroencephalography (EEG) is recorded during the neurofeedback treatment. Then its various components are extracted and fed to subjects using online feedback loop in the form of audio, video, or their combination.

—*Basic and Clinical Neuroscience*[91]

A neurological-based chiropractor will do a thorough assessment and recommend an appropriate schedule; frequently at first, then less often. Ask your doctor for a recommendation or do a Google search in your area. Chiropractic care may be more practical than massage therapy because most insurance companies will pay for this kind of treatment. In addition, some chiropractors also have massage therapists in their office.

Suggestion: Discuss the benefits of chiropractic therapy with your doctor to determine whether they feel this would be beneficial. If so, schedule an appointment for an initial assessment and follow their recommendations.

22

....

Traditional Chinese Medicine (TCM)

The main hurdle when it comes to treating mood issues is
it's a little like pain—you can feel it but we don't always know the cause.
Perhaps that's why TCM approaches make a lot of sense here, taking a
holistic look at as many variables and treatment options as possible.
—*Yin Yang You* by Aniong Xu, PhD & Mehmet Oz, MD

Traditional Chinese Medicine (TCM) is a natural way to treat many conditions, including anxiety and depression.

Traditional Chinese Medicine is a holistic system of healthcare that has been practiced for thousands of years in China and other parts of Asia. It views the body and mind as interconnected and influenced by the flow of vital energy (Qi) along pathways known as "meridians." TCM uses a combination of methods to identify and treat deficiencies and imbalances in the body.

—*Verywell Mind*[92]

TCM is recognized as a complementary therapy by the National Institutes of Health (NIH).[93] Associate professor Heidi Most at Maryland University of Integrative Health said several natural treatments can be useful in treating depression and anxiety, such as acupuncture, herbs, dietary therapy, Qi Gong, and Tai Chi.[94] She also said there is a disturbance to the *Shen* (our spirit) when we have anxiety or depression, which might lead to feelings of worthlessness or self-loathing. Also, our *qi* (energy) may be stuck so our emotions become stuck. TCM can help the qi move smoothly in the body and alleviate the feeling of being stuck.

Below is a brief description of each practice used in TCM to focus on treating and healing anxiety and depression.

1. **Qi Gong:** Gentle movements, breathing exercises, and meditation techniques with the goal of cultivating and balance qi, which can calm the mind, reduce stress, and promote emotional stability.

2. **Tai Chi:** Similar to Qi Gong but involves a more complex series of movements that work on the entire body; it combines slow, flowing movements with deep breathing and mental focus. This technique can promote relaxation, reduce anxiety, improve mood, and enhance cognitive function.

3. **Tuina massage:** A Chinese therapeutic massage, its focus is to stimulate acupressure points and manipulate the body's energy channels. Many studies showed improved sleep, relief of anxiety and depression, and regulated neurotransmitter levels.

4. **Feng Shui:** The practice of creating harmony and balance by arranging the environment to maximize the flow of qi (energy/life force). Furniture and decorations are placed to balance the *yin* and the *yang*. Numerous books and websites offer resources to learn more about this practice, but one is to incorporate blue tones—this can help with stress, anxiety, and depression (discussed further in Chapter 36).

5. **Moxibustion:** Burning dried mugwort leaves over certain acupuncture points stimulates circulation, promotes healing, and increases the flow of energy throughout the body. It should not be used if one is pregnant, has a mugwort allergy,

or has smoke sensitivity. You can do this at home or with a practitioner.

6. **Mindfulness and meditation:** These practices can decrease symptoms of depression, anxiety, worry, and anger (see Chapter 27).

7. **Dietary therapy:** Some foods have a significant impact on mental health; therefore, a balanced diet can support emotional well-being; fruits, vegetables, whole grains, and lean proteins are recommended.

8. **Herbs:** Discussed in the next chapter.

Suggestion: Talk to your doctor, psychologist and/or psychiatrist and do your own research to determine which practice would be most beneficial.

23

Traditional Chinese Medicine: Herbs

Chinese herbs have very real healing properties. There is a great deal of research on the clinical effectiveness of herbs used in Chinese medicine.
—Cynthia Chamberlain, DIPlAc, DIPlCH

Herbs have been used in TCM for over 3,000 years to treat many conditions, including depression and anxiety. One herbal blend for depression and PTSD is Xiao Yao San. A study on animals suggested that this herbal blend helps relieve depression by reducing neuroinflammation of the brain and spinal cord. Studies have shown that Xiao Yao San appears to improve symptoms of depression when taken alone or with an antidepressant and it has fewer side effects than antidepressants but do include headache, dizziness, and diarrhea.

Another herb that is used in TCM to treat depression is Yueju-Wan ethanol extract; a study found that it "alleviated the depressive symptoms in a rapid and lasting manner."[95] Gan Mai Da Zao decoction (GMDZ) is a third herbal blend used in TCM to treat depression. This is commonly used in TCM, but there are not a lot of studies to back up the effectiveness.

A variety of herbs are used in TCM to treat anxiety, such as ginkgo biloba that may be effective in relieving symptoms of anxiety when 480 mg per day is taken. Banxia-houpu decoction is a blend also used in TCM for severe anxiety but should be taken under the supervision of a healthcare provider. Other herbs that are beneficial for anxiety include chamomile, valerian, lavender, Galphimia glauca, passion-flower, kava, cannabidiol (CBD), and ashwagandha.

TCM herbs focus on healing the individual; Western medicine uses antidepressants and antianxiety medications that focus on masking symptoms. The herbs mentioned are available to buy without a prescription, but supplements are not regulated by the FDA so there is no guarantee that the product contains what the label says. Look for third-party testing and discuss herbs with your healthcare provider.

> **Suggestion:** Research the herbs above and discuss the benefits of taking them with your physician, psychiatrist, or psychologist.

24

....

Acupuncture, Acupressure, and Emotional Freedom Technique

The body is a self-healing system. When you cut your finger, it heals.
You don't need an advanced degree to be able to repair a wound . . .
In truth, we don't actually heal other people. We provide energy for other
people to heal themselves. Acupuncture works by freeing up a person's
own energy through the use of needles on meridians.
—Richard Gordon, *The Secret Nature of Matter*

Acupressure is one way to help your body fight back and balance itself in the face of the pressures of modern life. —Michael Reed Gach, *Acupressure's Potent Points: A Guide to Self-Care for Common Ailments*

Psychiatrists and other health care professionals are recommending acupuncture for depression and anxiety more often than ever before due to the many studies that show the benefits on mental health. An article entitled "Why Psychiatrists are Recommending Acupuncture to Their Patients" discusses four reasons psychiatrists are recommending acupuncture.[96]

1. **More research** supports acupuncture for mental health. Mayer gives details of three recent studies that showed levels of anxiety and depression were less with acupuncture than the control group and said that "acupuncture could be useful alongside medication."

2. **There are no side effects.** There are no side effects from acupuncture and the acupuncturist can treat the side effects of medications along with depression or anxiety.

3. **The results can be immediate.** "Since acupuncture moves qi, blood, and fluids, which can reduce inflammation and thereby reduce pain, you regularly see pain reduction immediately after treatment—not just from the endorphin release but from the reduction of inflammation. According to researchers, chronic inflammation may be linked to depression." Mayer stated that a person needs to get a treatment at least once a week to be effective.

4. **More people are seeking help for their mental health.** Seeking help has increased significantly since the start of the COVID-19 pandemic.

Acupuncture and acupressure are similar techniques used in TCM as they both stimulate the meridians to improve blood flow. They move chi/life force energy through the meridians that support the main

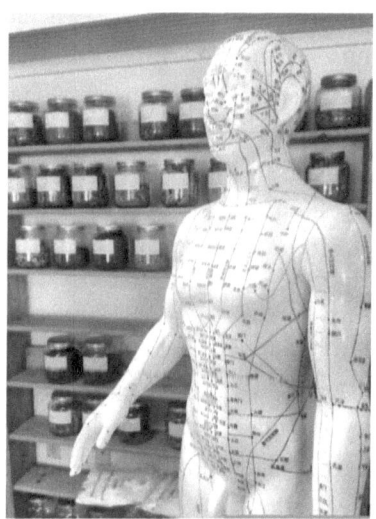

Meridians in the body

organs in the body, making them stronger. Twelve principal meridians and eight additional meridians are divided into yin and yang groups. While acupuncture uses small needles, acupressure uses fingertips. It is generally thought that acupuncture is more effective because it can stimulate the acupoint more strongly. Currently, there is not enough evidence to support acupuncture and acupressure as a treatment for depression, but some studies suggest that when used in conjunction with medication, depression symptoms are significantly reduced.

The meridian points of focus are inside the wrists and between the eyes and ears. These techniques are administered by a qualified practitioner. A technique known as the emotional freedom technique (EFT), or tapping, was created by Gary Craig and can be administered on your own. According to Healthline, "EFT is an alternative treatment for physical pain and emotional distress" and involves five steps[97]:

1. **Identify the issue:** Choose one issue to focus on.

2. **Rate the intensity:** Rate the intensity of your feelings from 0–10.

3. **Setting up:** Find a phrase to repeat that addresses the issue and self-acceptance (such as, "Even though my partner left me, I deeply and completely accept myself").

4. **Tapping sequence:** Start with tapping the side of your hand while repeating the phrase you created for three cycles. Then tap the following, in order: eyebrow, side of eye, beneath eye, under your nose, on your chin, at the place your collarbone begins, beneath your arm, and the top of your head. Each time you tap on an area, repeat your phrase. Go through the complete sequence two to three times.

5. **Testing the results:** Using the 0–10 scale, rate how you feel. If it is not a 0, keep repeating the steps until you can rate a 0.

It may sound difficult to do but it isn't. I learned how to do it properly through YouTube videos and have been using this technique for years. Discuss this technique with your doctor as certain people should not use this method, including those who have an automatic implantable cardioverter-defibrillator (AICD) or suffer from psychosis or delusions.

Suggestion: Start with EFT by watching YouTube videos to learn the technique. Also talk to your doctor about the benefits of acupuncture or acupressure.

~ VI ~
Introduction: Spirit

We are not in control of what happens around us,
but we remain in control of what happens inside us.
—Unknown

I love this quote because many people look outside themselves for help with their feelings, but we are the only ones who can make the changes, and we need to be aligned with our spirit to allow these changes to happen. A definition of spirit is "the principle of life, feeling, thought, and action in humans, regarded as a distinct entity separate from the body, and commonly held to be separable in existence from the body; the spiritual part of humans as distinct from the physical body."[98] This section of the book explains that our spirit and everything else in the universe, is energy, and energy is simply vibration. Numerous ways to raise our vibration to align with spirit are discussed in this section.

The first chapter explains energy and vibrations; the others offer ways to raise our vibration: prayer, meditation, music, crystals, laughter, nature, sunshine, animals, smudging, subliminal messages, aromatherapy, Epsom salt baths, colors, and Feng Shui. There are many other spiritual practices, but this will give you some direction on where to start.

Keep in mind that there is a connection between mind, body, and spirit, so there are other chapters in the mind and body sections that are also spiritual. Research shows spirituality can benefit the body and the mind, especially when directed with intentional practices and that spiritual exercises help us decrease negative emotions, find meaning, and strengthen relationships with others.[99]

> **Suggestion:** First read the chapter on energy to get a better understanding of the importance of raising our vibration. Then read the remaining chapters and focus on the practices that you resonate with the most. Choose one or two practices to incorporate into your daily life.

25

....

Energy

We begin to achieve higher frequencies by recognizing
the pattern of "like attracts like." More than just a saying,
this is an energetic law. Frequencies are attracted to similar frequencies.
We resonate at a higher frequency when we raise our vibration,
and therefore, attract higher level experiences.
—Caroline A. Shearer,
Raise Your Vibration: Tips and Tools for a High-Frequency Life

Energy is such an important topic because everything in the universe is made up of energy, and all energy has a vibration. In 2006, Rhonda Byrne published *The Secret*, in which she explained the law of attraction.[100] Reading this book was the beginning of my interest in energy and vibration, on what this powerful law of the universe can do for us. Since then, I have read dozens of books on the subject and learned tools to raise my vibration to attract what I want in my life. The basic principle of "like attracts like" says that you must become the energy to attract similar energy.

One of the most powerful authors I have read on this subject is David R. Hawkins who has written several books explaining the "Map of Consciousness" that he developed.[101] He outlines the levels of energy that humankind experiences, from the lowest level of shame (20) to the highest level of enlightenment (700–1,000). This numerical value is determined through muscle testing, a technique of applying pressure to a muscle when a statement is given. The response will be a yes or not yes (no) answer. If the statement is true, the muscle remains strong, but if the statement is not true, the muscle goes weak. Without going into too much detail, if a person is depressed or anxious, they are vibrating at a low frequency so it is critical to raise their vibration up on the scale of the Map of Consciousness.

Map of Consciousness
from *Power vs. Force* by David Hawkins

God-view	Life-view	Level	Log	Emotion	Process
Self	is	Enlightenment	700-1,000 ↑	Ineffable	Pure Consciousness
All-Being	Perfect	Peace	600 ↑	Bliss	Illumination
One	Complete	Joy	540 ↑	Serenity	Transfiguration
Loving	Benign	Love	500 ↑	Reverence	Revelation
Wise	Meaningful	Reason	400 ↑	Understanding	Abstraction
Merciful	Harmonious	Acceptance	350 ↑	Forgiveness	Transcendence
Inspiring	Hopeful	Willingness	310 ↑	Optimism	Intention
Enabling	Satisfactory	Neutrality	250 ↑	Trust	Release
Permitting	Feasible	Courage	200 ⬦	Affirmation	Empowerment
Indifferent	Demanding	Pride	175 ↓	Scorn	Inflation
Vengeful	Antagonistic	Anger	150 ↓	Hate	Aggression
Denying	Disappointing	Desire	125 ↓	Craving	Enslavement
Punitive	Frightening	Fear	100 ↓	Anxiety	Withdrawal
Disdainful	Tragic	Grief	75 ↓	Regret	Despondency
Condemning	Hopeless	Apathy	50 ↓	Despair	Abdication
Vindictive	Evil	Guilt	30 ↓	Blame	Destruction

At the level of shame, a person has the core belief that they are not good enough (associated with depression); that causes energetic and physical stagnation that results in "blocked" energy. Many YouTube videos talk more about this, but here are some ways to raise your vibration, which are discussed in this book.

1. Reiki
2. Crystal healing
3. Sound healing
4. Meditation and mindful breathing
5. Psych K
6. Prayer
7. Gratitude
8. Yoga
9. Nature
10. Tapping
11. Exercise and movement
12. Kindness
13. Positive self-affirmations
14. Surrounding yourself with positive people
15. Music
16. Proper nutrition
17. Adequate sleep
18. Spiritual mind treatment
19. Sunlight
20. Avoiding drugs and alcohol
21. Grounding
22. Forgiveness
23. Volunteering
24. Acupuncture and acupressure
25. Cranial sacral therapy

26. Massage and aromatherapy

27. Chiropractic therapy

28. Drinking plenty of water

29. Psychotherapy

30. Laughter

31. Pranic healing

32. Shamanic healing

33. Chi Kung

34. Chi Quong

35. Subliminal recordings

36. Colors

37. Feng Shui

38. Smudging

39. Epsom salt bath

40. Essential oils

Suggestion: Try several ways to raise your vibrational frequency to see which ones resonate with you and focus on those chapters first.

26

....

Prayer

Never underestimate the power of prayer! Constant prayer,
with full conviction, without loss of hope, really does create miracles.
—Ritu Ghatourey

Prayer is a powerful tool we all have access to, and it doesn't matter what your religious beliefs are; all religions practice some form of prayer. It is our communication with God, the Divine, the Almighty, or the multitude of other names that can be used. *Psychology Today* states that prayer is not just helpful for those without mental illness; it also has a positive impact on people who are lonely and those recovery from mental illness.[102]

Types of prayers include praise for God, prayers of petition (asking for what we need, including forgiveness), prayers of intersession (asking for what others need), and prayers of thanksgiving (for what God has done for us or given us).

Prayer chains are when a group of people pray for a specific person or reason for a pre-determined amount of time; additionally, there are global prayer chains. There is no right way to pray as prayers may be said aloud or silently, with our eyes open or closed, sitting, kneeling, or standing. Many people wonder if their prayers are heard and answered by God. A way to evaluate this is if we feel it in our hearts and we get a feeling of peace and calmness. But what if our prayers are not answered?

If our prayers do not seem to be answered, it doesn't mean it is a punishment from God. Sometimes we are praying for something that is not what we need, and God becomes silent as a way for us to have a heart-check and realize we are praying with wrong motives. Over 50 Bible verses offer prayers for healing.[103] Below are some of the key scriptures in the Bible.

- 1 Peter 2:24 *By His wounds you have been healed.*

- Isaiah 40:29 *He gives strength to the weary and increases the power of the weak.*

- Psalm 147:3 *He heals the brokenhearted and binds up their wounds.*

- James 5:14–15 *The prayer offered in faith will make the sick person well.*

- Jeremiah 17:14 *Heal me, Lord, and I will be healed; save me and I will be saved.*

Miracles are said to have occurred using prayer. Canonization in the Catholic Church declares someone a saint after they have performed two or more miracles. An article[104] sums up the canonization process as "a miracle almost always is the spontaneous and lasting remission of a serious, life-threatening medical condition. The healing must have taken place in ways that the best-informed scientific knowledge cannot account for and follow prayers to the holy person." Some well-known figures who performed miracles, besides Jesus, were Mother Teresa of Calcutta and St. Francis of Assisi.

The prayer of St. Francis of Assisi:
> Lord, make me an instrument of Your Peace
> Where there is hatred, let me sow love
> Where there is injury, pardon
> Where there is doubt, faith
> Where there is despair, hope
> Where there is darkness, light
> And where there is sadness, joy.

Litany of St. Francis of Assisi:
> Lord, have mercy on us. Christ, have mercy on us.
> Lord, have mercy on us. Christ, hear us.
> Christ, graciously hear us.
> God, the Father of Heaven, Have mercy on us.
> God the Son, the Redeemer of the world, Have mercy on us.
> God the Holy Spirit, Have mercy on us.
> Holy Trinity, One God, Have mercy on us.

Mother Teresa of Calcutta's favorite prayer:
> Dear Jesus, help me to spread Thy fragrance everywhere I go. Flood my soul with Thy spirit and love. Penetrate and possess my whole being so utterly that all my life may only be a radiance of Thine. Shine through me and be so in me that every soul I come in contact with may feel Thy presence in my soul. Let them look up and see no longer me, but only Jesus. Stay with me and then I shall begin to shine as you shine, so to shine as to be a light to others. Amen.[105]

Another form of prayer is a spiritual mind treatment, an affirmative prayer established by Ernest Holmes, who founded the Religious Science movement in 1927.[106] This type of prayer is a five-step process in which the person giving the prayer has an absolute knowing that what they are praying for is already done. I know from personal experience that this form of prayer works as I have had my prayers answered many times. A basic description of the steps:

1. **Recognition** God is all there is.
2. **Unification** I am one with God.
3. **Realization** I accept and embody my good.
4. **Thanksgiving** I give thanks, knowing the healing has already occurred.
5. **Release** I let go and let God.

During my training to become a Science of Mind practitioner, I gave many people spiritual mind treatments. Below is a sample of one of many successful treatments; a woman in her late 60s had plans to hike to 10,000 feet to release her husband's ashes. She wanted prayers to hike successfully to that elevation and for all her family members to feel comfortable emotionally.

Treatment for Janice
There is one Divine Source that runs in and through everything seen and unseen. This Divine Source we call many things—God, Love, First Cause, Omnipotent. In God, all things are possible. There is nothing that cannot be achieved when God is recognized as all-powerful. This God energy that is present is present everywhere, it is present in me, it is present in Janice, and it is present in every other person. Since God is present in everyone, we have all the power available to us. Because this is true, I know the truth that Janice, as the matri arch of her family, knows exactly how to scatter Ben's ashes. She is confident in her ability to listen to Spirit and be guided by Spirit. She trusts that Spirit will guide her each step of the way and knows that whatever she is called to say and do is

for the highest good for her and her family. Janice is focused and courageous because she listens to Spirit and trust in It. She knows when, and how to scatter Ben's ashes. She trusts in the guidance she receives from Spirit. She is physically, mentally, and emotionally strong. Her body can hike, climb, and acclimate to high elevations. She hikes in Yosemite with ease, grace, and glory. Knowing this truth for Janice, I release my word into the law, knowing that it is done, and for this I give abundant gratitude. And so it is!

The benefits of prayer are numerous, but the idea is to pray to God however you choose. Prayer is beneficial for our mental health and miracles do happen.

Suggestion: Start a daily practice of prayer and consider a prayer chain.

27

Meditation

Where there is peace and meditation, there is neither anxiety nor doubt.
—St. Francis De Sales

The importance of meditation is becoming more widely accepted due to its many benefits as evidenced by the annual World Meditation Day on May 21 and the annual United Nations World Meditation Day on December 21.[107] How does meditation affect the structure of brain?[108] Two regions of the brain have been linked to depression; one is the medial prefrontal cortex (mPFC) that becomes hyperactive in people with depression, the other region is amygdala or "fear center" that is responsible for the fight-or-flight response. Meditation has been found to be helpful because it breaks the connection between these two regions of the brain associated with depression. Healthline.com states that meditation is helpful for reducing stress and anxiety, may enhance your mood, and can help with sleep.[109]

Several types of meditation are beneficial for people who are depressed or anxious: loving-kindness, mindfulness, mindful-ness-based cognitive therapy, transcendental, yoga, visualization, chanting and walking meditation, pranayama, The Moses Code[110] (based on the book by James F. Twyman), Psych K[111] (originated by Rob Williams), and Wayne Dyer's CD series called Meditations for Manifesting.[112] YouTube has many guided meditations that can be useful as well. Another resource is the application Insight Timer with a variety of guided meditations.[113] Through meditation, the mind is focused on one thing to overcome negative feelings and emotions are associated with depression. Here is a seven-step guide offered by NHS for beginners:

1. **Set aside some time.** Get in the habit of meditating for 20 minutes twice a day, once in the morning and once before going to bed.

2. **Find a comfortable place.** Sit in a comfortable, upright position.

3. **Bring mindfulness into meditation.** Close your eyes and focus on the present moment by being consciously aware of your senses, such as what you hear, feel, or smell.

4. **Start your meditation.** Breathe in while saying to yourself "breathe in," and your belly should expand slightly. Breathe out while saying "breathe out," and your belly should go in slightly.

5. **The challenge is focusing the mind.** It is normal to have a wandering mind; notice when it is distracted by a thought and bring it back to focus on breathing.

6. **Get the hang of meditation.** Meditation takes practice; if you have intruding thoughts, acknowledge them and gently focus your mind on breathing again. Breathing naturally can be difficult when focusing on the balance between circular breath and natural breath. It just takes practice. Don't judge your meditation practice. There is no right or wrong way.

7. **Bring your meditation to a close.** When finishing your meditation, stop focusing on your breath but stay seated with your eyes closed for a few minutes. Then open your eyes and calmly transition to the next part of your day.[114]

One meditation practice that I used regularly as an elementary school teacher was from the website GoNoodle.[115] I felt their guided meditations helped the children calm down and lower anxiety. Introducing children to meditation at an early age can set them up for a lifetime meditation practice. Healthychildren.org[116] has guidelines for meditation length by age group; for preschool children, a few minutes a day is appropriate, for grade school children, three to ten minutes a day is appropriate, and for teens and adults, the range is from five minutes to 45 minutes a day.

Hopefully, insurance companies will soon cover transcendental meditation (TM) and make it more affordable. Meditate America, the David Lynch Foundation wants to make TM available to those most in need of it: first responders such as healthcare workers, firefighters, and law enforcement; veterans, inner-city students, survivors of domestic violence, and adults and teens battling substance use disorder.[117]

Benefits of TM include reducing stress, improving sleep, controlling anxiety, reducing blood pressure, increasing productivity, enhancing mental clarity, and cultivating stronger relationships.[118] Since TM is effective in reducing chronic stress, the root cause of 90% of all illnesses—it creates better health and well-being. There are many different forms of meditation but TM "is a process of automatic self-transcending, allowing the practitioner to experience a field of calm deep within."[119]

A video about the benefits of TM presented by Bob Roth, CEO, and the actor Hugh Jackman is very informative; it gives an example regarding veterans and the suicide rates of first responders (their number one cause of death). Studies have shown that TM is effective in reducing this number.

Suggestion: Choose a meditation practice or find a YouTube-guided video meditation and become comfortable using it. Then meditate twice daily for 20 minutes.

28

....

Music

Great music is a great remedy for depression,
but you have to drink it in with your heart and mind.
—Debasish Mrihda

Music—which helps reduce depression—includes the following benefits:

1. Listening to classical music helps improve sleep quality.

2. Happy music can lift your mood.

3. Calming music can reduce stress.

Music therapy, along with other therapies, can be used to reduce depression. A music therapist uses customized music to help people understand and process their emotions, but you can find music on your own. Look for music that plays 60 beats per minute for a relaxed, conscious mind. This tempo activates the alpha brainwaves that can induce calmness, lower stress, reduce anxiety, decrease depression, increase creativity, and enhance your ability to absorb new information. I have included several songs and artists below.

1. *My Girl* (LP version), Otis Redding

2. *Love is All*, The Wild Hunt

3. *Landslide*, Fleetwood Mac

4. *Try a Little Tenderness*, Otis Redding

5. *Simple Man*, Lynyrd Skynyrd

6. *Desperado* (2013 Remaster), Eagles

7. *Turn the Page*, Metallica

8. *Mustang Sally*, Wilson Picket

Music that is 432 hertz (Hz) relaxes the brain but note that certain music has the opposite effect. Studies suggest a correlation between music that expresses negative emotions and an increase in anxiety. Sad music is particularly harmful to adolescents because of the ruminating negative thoughts they might be having.

The abstract "The Effects of Different Types of Music on Mood, Tension, and Mental Clarity" is particularly informative.[120] This study included 144 subjects who listened to four different types of music for 15 minutes and completed a profile before and after. Grunge music was found to be the most harmful as it increased hostility, sadness, tension, and fatigue, decreased caring, relaxation, mental clarity, and vigor. Grunge music can be defined as "rock music incorporating elements of punk rock and heavy metal."[121] The most beneficial music to listen to was designer music; subjects demonstrated more caring, relaxation, mental clarity, and vigor. Designer music is music created to have a specific effect on the listener. The last two types of music were classical and New Age, which showed mixed results.

Suggestion: Listen to music that has 60 beats per minute or designer music daily; both can be found on Amazon and other websites. Avoid sad music and grunge music.

29

Vibrational Sound Therapy

Life as manifested is vibration. Vibration is motion; therefore,
all life is in motion. Harmony of vibration unites life forms.
—Dorinne Davis

Let's start with a definition of sound healing since not everyone is familiar with this. The Sound Healing Academy defines it as "a powerful therapy that combines different healing sounds, music, and sound healing instruments to improve our multidimensional well-being by creating a beautiful experience where all layers of our luminous energy field (body, mind, soul, spirit) are awakened gently and lovingly."[122]

Sound healing is an effective way to trigger our relaxation response and may relieve chronic stress. A variety of instruments can be used, such as Tibetan and crystal singing bowls, gongs, drums, and tuning forks. Astute Counseling and Wellness[123] describes a few:

1. **Singing Bowls:** Usually made of metal or crystal, they produce resonant sounds when struck or played with a mallet.

2. **Tuning Forks:** These produce specific frequencies, and when placed on the body, stimulate energetic balance.

3. **Gongs:** These have powerful, multidimensional sounds in which vibrations can penetrate deep into the body.

4. **Drums:** The rhythmic beat of drums has been used for centuries to facilitate healing.

Sandy LaBianco Brown from Rush University System for Health[124] lists some benefits of vibrational sound therapy:

1. Reduces stress
2. Reduces pain
3. Eases blockages and tension
4. Reduces depression
5. Improves sleep
6. Boosts creativity
7. Improves concentration
8. Balances energy fields (aura) and chakras
9. Lowers blood pressure

LaBianco Brown said that soothing sounds and vibration on a relaxed body affects the body at a cellular level. Stress creates an unhealthy energy flow, but vibrational sound therapy opens the energy flow to move back toward a healthy alignment. Some instruments are placed directly on the body, while other instruments are played above the body, creating a physical vibration throughout the body. During this time, the practitioner is focusing on spiritual and energetic connections. According to Vibrational Sound Therapist Crissy Campbell, counseling and vibrational sound therapy go together. She explained that having a vibrational sound therapy session immediately following counseling is beneficial; a lot of emotions arise during counseling can be released from the body through vibrational sound therapy, helping patients process their emotions.[125]

A form of vibration sound therapy is a sound bath, basically a form of meditation that uses unique instruments that create waves of soothing sounds that may help with stress and depression symptoms. While more research is needed, some have experienced positive effects on their mental health. Like all the other holistic approaches discussed, this is an adjunct therapy to go along with counseling and/ or medication.

To find a qualified practitioner, start with Google search for someone qualified in vibrational sound therapy or crystal bowl sound. Then check for their credentials, certificates, and training.

> **Suggestion:** Search your area local to find a qualified vibrational sound healer and discuss the healing options.

30

....

Reiki

Reiki is love, love is wholeness, wholeness is balance,
balance is well-being, well-being is freedom from disease.
—Dr. Mikao Usui

Reiki (pronounced *ray*-key) is a form of energy healing discovered by
Mikao Usui in Japan in the late 1800s; *rei* means spiritual wisdom and
ki means life energy. A Reiki treatment involves a practitioner placing
their hands on or above a person, and through a series of hand place-
ments, they become a conduit to transfer this universal life force energy

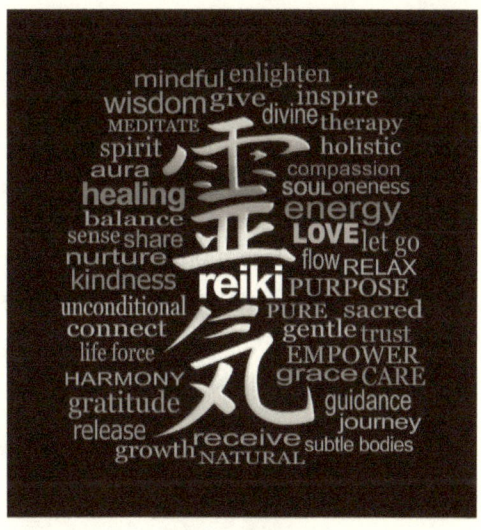

Reiki symbol

to that person. Everyone has ki (universal life force energy) flowing through their bodies through pathways called *chakras* that regulate *meridians*—channels that our energy flows through. Chakras can become blocked and the energy in the surrounding area becomes stagnant and blocked. For well-being in the body, the energy needs to flow freely. A Reiki practitioner channels the Reiki energy to unblock the chakras.

While Reiki was not widely accepted by the scientific and medical communities in the past, it is becoming more mainstream, and some insurance companies will cover the treatments. Proponents of Reiki (and a small number of studies) have shown that Reiki can have positive effects on an individual, such as reducing anxiety and depression.

The Reiki Healing Association[126] cites many studies that have shown Reiki decreases stress and anxiety. It also promotes emotional balance, improves sleep and reduces insomnia, supports trauma recovery, and enhances self-awareness and mindfulness. The five principles that encourage practitioners to cultivate a mindful approach to life are:

1. Just for today, I will not be angry.

2. Just for today, I will not worry.

3. Just for today, I will be grateful.

4. Just for today, I will do my work honestly.

5. Just for today, I will be kind to every living thing.

This treatment should be used along with other treatments such as counseling. To find a Reiki practitioner in your area you can do an easy Google search.

> **Suggestion:** Find a Reiki master in your area and schedule an appointment to discuss possible treatment.

31

Healing Crystals

*Crystals channel energy. They can focus, store, transmit, and transmute
this energy and it can be used for beneficial healing and energizing effects.*
—Philip Permutt

Crystals have been used for their healing properties around the world
for thousands of years, but there is no scientific evidence to support
that. However, crystals vibrate at a much higher level (32,768 Hz) than
humans (7.5 Hz). As discussed earlier, someone who is depressed is
vibrating at a very low frequency, so raising their vibration is beneficial.
When we are exposed to crystals, it raises our vibrational frequency.

Crystals carry a specific vibrational frequency, a dominant oscil-
latory rate (DOR), that can be raised or lowered. Since crystals have
a higher vibration than humans, they can raise our vibrational frequency, called entrainment. According to crystal healer Jessica Garcia,
humans are basically chaotic because we are emotional beings; crystals
are stable, and their frequency does not change so they can stabilize
the chaos within us. "The stable frequency of the crystal will automat-
ically calm the chaos, resulting in clearing any blocks and creating
balance."[127]

Specific crystals have specific healing properties so it is best to
choose the ones that would be most beneficial. Clear quartz is thought
of as the universal metaphysical stone or the "feel better" crystal and
is a great crystal to start with for channeling energy and helping with

any condition. Another powerful crystal is amethyst, a form of quartz with a purple color due to manganese and iron inclusions. It helps with emotional and mental balance. If someone is dealing with anxiety and depression, it is best to treat the anxiety first.

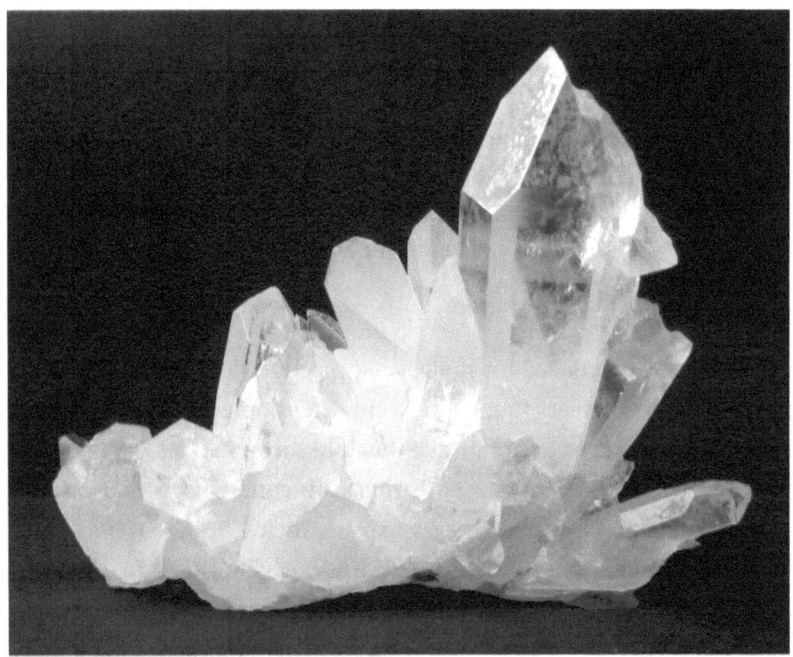

Clear quartz—a master healer

Anxiety:

1. **Amethyst:** Soft calming energy that soothes irritability, balances mood swings, and helps with anger, fear, and anxiety.

2. **Malachite:** Helps depression and manic depression. Works well when paired with lepidolite.

3. **Lepidolite:** Lithium-bearing mineral used as an antianxiety medication.

4. **Black tourmaline:** Has grounding properties and absorbs negative energy. It also creates a protective shield from electromagnetic frequencies (EMF) around someone and is soothing.

5. **Rose quartz:** Associated with love and emotional healing and promotes self-love, self-acceptance, and compassion.

Depression:

1. **Amethyst**

2. **Lepidolite**

3. **Citrine:** Yellow to brownish-yellow quartz that promotes joy and optimism. It also helps with insomnia.

4. **Carnelian:** Helps with anger, envy, fear, rage, sorrow, confusion, and jealousy.

Crystals can be placed nearby, held, placed on the body, meditated with, worn, carried in a pocket, or made into elixirs with crystals and water: place specific crystals in water (best to use distilled or mineral water), cover, and refrigerate overnight.[128] A caution about elixirs: Some crystals are toxic, so it is best to place them *around* the water unless you have researched the specific crystal. Just placing crystals around the water will give the same benefits as placing them in the water.

When working with crystals, ensure you cleanse them regularly as they absorb energy from people and the environment. One of the easiest ways to clean is to run water over them for about a minute and use your fingers to wash them gently. (Caution: Crystals ending in -*ite*, such as lepidolite, should not be submerged in water.) After washing the crystals, place them in the sun to dry; be careful with quartz because sunlight can cause a fire risk, and some crystals may fade in sunlight. Another method is to dust them gently with a soft brush. If you have a geode, you can place your crystal inside it to cleanse. Sound cleansing can also be used by using singing bowls, tuning forks, bells, and chanting. YouTube videos have music for cleansing crystals. When there is a new moon or a full moon, you can leave the crystals outside.

> **Suggestion:** If you are new to crystals, start with a clear quartz; carry it with you and keep it next to your bed when sleeping. Find an expert in crystal healing and see them regularly.

32

·············

Laughter

We don't laugh because we're happy, we're happy because we laugh.
—William James

Always laugh when you can. It is cheap medicine.
—Poet Lord Byron

There are many benefits of laughter, according to William F. Fry who pioneered the field of gelotology (the study of laughter), there is much value in laughter; not only does it benefit us physically, but also mentally. Laughter causes a release of mood boosting chemicals including endorphins.[129] Your brain releases fewer stress hormones, reducing the symptoms of depression. While we can laugh when we are alone, we laugh 30 times more when with other people. Sophie Scott, a British cognitive neuroscientist describes this as "social emotion."[130] there are many ways to you can incorporate laughter into life by developing the seven "humor habits" devised by Paul McGhee in his book *Humor as Survival Training for a Stressed-Out World*.[131] Surround yourself with humor by watching comedies, comedians, short funny YouTube clips, and reading funny jokes. Try to find more joy in whatever you are doing. Be intentional about laughing more and look for humor in everyday events.

More formal practices to laugh more with humor, such as laughter yoga, has been shown to reduce depression and loneliness.[132] A medical doctor from India, Madan Kataria, discovered in 1995 that when someone laughed for whatever reason, others began to laugh too. Laughter yoga is still around today and incorporates playful movement and exercises.

Suggestion: Incorporate laughter daily by watching comedies, comedians, or short funny YouTube clips.

33

....

Nature

When we spend time outside in beautiful places, a part of our brain
called the subgenual prefrontal cortex quiets down, and this is the part of
the brain that is associated with negative self-reported rumination.
—Florence Williams

There are so many benefits to being in nature that it is worth focusing
on. Many studies have shown benefits to brain activity, as measured
by electroencephalogram (EEG) and magnetic resonance imaging
(MRI). Activity in the brain is affected positively, such as lower activation in the amygdala and decreased blood flow in the prefrontal cortex.
The subgenual prefrontal cortex (SGPFC) is the area of the brain that
involves emotional regulation and has been associated with bipolar
disorder. While there is no definitive amount of time that is needed,
two hours a week is most beneficial for self-reported well-being.

Nature has played a role in healing for many years. For example, in
357 BC, Hippocrates designed a hospital with a garden to help patients
heal. In the 1980s, Japan's experiments with nature, *shinrin-yoku* or
forest-bathing, showed measurable changes in stress hormones. The
process of forest-bathing is to walk slowly through the forest, taking in the environment through all your senses. Qing Li, a Japanese
medical doctor and researcher, wrote the book *Forest-Bathing: How
Trees Can Help You Find Health and Happiness* in which he reports
some disturbing statistics about the amount of time Americans spend

indoors.[133] According to *Time* magazine, too much time spent indoors can fuel anxiety and insomnia; the body's circadian rhythm regulated by sunlight affects sleep, mood, and energy levels. When the circadian rhythm is disrupted by erratic sleep (jet lag, night workers, etc.), there is a link to depression. *Time* also reported that a series of experiments conducted at the University of Rochester demonstrated a 40% increase in vitality as a result of spending time outdoors in nature.[134] If you are interested in learning more about shinrin-yoku, Dr. Li's book is available on Amazon.com.

While forest-bathing is one method of improving mental well-being, just being in nature has benefits. According to Andrew Avitt, green spaces are good for our physical health because they support an active, healthy lifestyle that is associated with increasing life expectancy, better sleep, and a reduced risk of cancer. He speaks about the benefits on our mental health also:

> There are many mental wellness benefits associated with being outside in green spaces, such as lower risk of depression and faster psychological stress recovery. Studies have shown that being in nature can restore and strengthen our mental capacities, increasing focus and attention.[135]

While green spaces are good for our mental health, there is still air pollution to think about; it is linked to a higher risk of depression and anxiety. A review of 100 studies revealed that 73% of them found mental health symptoms related to outdoor air pollution because air pollution affects the regions of the brain that regulate emotions. Parks have basically the same air quality as cities, so when discussing nature, think of the beach or the forest.

There are things you can do though when outside to avoid exposure to pollutants such as staying away from burning wood, vehicle exhaust, and tobacco smoke, and wearing a mask outdoors. If it is not possible to go to the beach or mountains where the air is cleaner, it is still beneficial for our mental health to be outside, just take steps to avoid pollutants.

Suggestion: Spend as much time in nature as you can free from distractions such as technology and focus on appreciating natural beauty through your senses.

34

Sunshine

Keep your face to the sunshine and you cannot see the shadows.
It's what the sunflowers do.
—Helen Keller

Healthline addresses the importance of sunshine on our well-being and says that when we do not get enough sunlight, serotonin in our brain is decreased, which can lead to depression. Research also states that regular exposure to sunshine can elevate your mood and reduce sadness because sunlight releases the mood boosting chemical serotonin into the brain. "Low levels of serotonin are associated with a higher risk of major depression with seasonal patterns (formally known as seasonal affective disorder, or SAD)."[136]

Light therapy, or photo therapy, is one way to receive the benefits of the sunshine while staying inside. A light therapy box with an intensity of 10,000 lux—about the same light intensity as the sun—can stimulate the brain's ability to make serotonin with just 30 minutes daily use. There is a wide range of light therapy boxes on Amazon.com.

Another way to increase serotonin levels without being in the sun is to take 1,000 IUs daily of vitamin D3 but know it takes several weeks for the vitamin D levels to rise. Along with vitamin D3, vitamin K2 should also be taken; it helps your body transport vitamin D3 to your bones and teeth.

Suggestion: Get 15–20 minutes of sunshine daily, use a light therapy box, or take 1,000 IUs of vitamin D3.

35

Animals

Happiness is a warm puppy.
—Charles M. Shulz

Being around animals has a positive effect on our mental health and one way to do that is to have a pet. A considerable benefit of owning a pet is that they give us unconditional love. Interacting with pets can lower our cortisol levels (the stress hormone), reduce anxiety, depression, loneliness, and boost our mood. Pet therapy, or animal-assisted therapy, is for a person who needs the emotional support of an animal outside of home. A healthcare provider can write a letter to allow a person to take their pet, usually a dog, to public places that don't normally allow pets. An emotional support animal (ESA) does not need to wear anything identifying it in most states and does not require special training. Studies have shown the correlation between the use of an emotional support animal and improvements in mental health.[137]

A 2020 international study by the Assistance Dog Center showed that "all participants reported that their quality of life had improved as a result of having an ESA dog, and almost all reported that having an ESA dog increased their feelings of security, independence, and energy, and helped improve their sleep."[138] Another study conducted in the UK during the COVID-19 pandemic found similar results; almost 90% of people who had companion animals reported receiving considerable support from their animal. South Navato Animal Hospital lists some advantages of companion animals.[139]

1. **Boosts your physical activity:** Walking your dog is one way to boost your physical activity and is beneficial for mental health.

2. **Provides companionship:** Not only are pets good company but caring for an animal shifts focus to the animal from your personal challenges.

3. **Facilitates social connections:** Being around other pet owners can help you build new connections.

4. **Enhances daily organization:** For someone who is depressed and doesn't want to get out of bed, a pet can be a good motivator.

5. **Reduces anxiety:** The emotional support from an animal can reduce stress levels.

Animals have been shown to provide many benefits to our mental health, but they are not a cure-all for mental health issues; they are just one more way of helping people cope with problems. A person with mental health issues should work with their medical provider.

Suggestion: Get an emotional support animal to take outside the home with you or get a pet that can be a companion at home.

36

Additional Ways to Raise Your Vibration

Everything in life is vibration.
—Albert Einstein

As demonstrated in the section on energy, there are numerous ways to raise your vibration—and this is critical when dealing with anxiety and depression. While I've devoted whole chapters to standard practices, other practices beneficial for overall mental health are not as common; here are a few.

Shamanic healing is a religious practice used mostly by Indigenous and tribal societies. A shaman heals a person by communicating with the spirit world (the collective unconscious). According to their beliefs, psychological issues such as anxiety and depression have a spiritual component and may respond well to Shamanic healing.

Smudging, an ancient Native American ritual, involves burning sage to dissipate negative energy and improve mood. The steps below are from Spirit and Muse that also has a YouTube video to help you.[140]

1. Light the thick end of the sage (dried) and blow out the fire once it produces smoke. The smoke is what does the clearing.

2. Start in the corner of the room and move the smoke up and down. You can use a feather or your hand to fan the smoke.

3. Move to each of the corners in the room.

4. Once you've saged the corners of the room, move to the center (and the rest of the room), moving the smoke over any furniture and electronics.

5. Once you feel like you've done enough in that room, move to the next room and repeat the steps above. Start on the lowest level (basement or ground floor) of your home and work your way up to the top level.

6. As you are saging each room, remember to show gratitude to the Great Spirit for helping you clear your energy and your space. Repeat your mantra as you move to different areas of your home.

7. Once you've done each room, sage the entrance to your home by moving the smoke around the door frame.

Smudging can also be used on yourself or someone else to dissipate negative energy and improve mood. Before you begin smudging, have your mantra prepared. It can be anything you choose but here are a couple of examples: *Release any negativity into the light. May this space be a place of love, peace, and joy.*

I have found playing **subliminal recordings** when I am sleeping immensely helpful in raising my vibrational level. A subliminal recording is music or other pleasing sounds such as ocean waves or rain that have positive affirmations through the music that you cannot hear consciously. This works on your unconscious mind to slowly make changes. These recordings can be found on YouTube or Amazon.

Aromatherapy is another practice I use daily to relieve anxiety. An essential oil is extracted from bark, flowers, leaves, stems, roots, and other parts of plants. When added to water in a diffuser and turned on, the disc vibrates and creates ultrasonic waves that break the oil into microscopic particles and are released in a fine mist that is inhaled. As with smudging, this practice should be used as an ancillary treatment.

Studies support the use of essential oils for anxiety—such as lavender, sweet orange, yuzu, bergamot, chamomile, rosemary, sage, Spanish sage, lavender and Damascus rose combined, and lavender, ylang-ylang, and neroli combined.

Soaking in an **Epsom salt bath** is also helpful for reducing anxiety. Adding two cups of Epsom salt to a warm bath and relaxing in the water promotes relaxation, reducing anxiety and depression. When I was working full time, I took Epsom salt baths frequently at the end of the day and found it helpful in reducing stress.

The **colors** you surround yourself with also have an impact on your mental health. Colors that invoke emotional arousal are red, gray, and dark blue; some colors induce anxiety, such as red and orange. Colors for reducing stress and anxiety include pistachio green, sky blue, purple, violet, lavender, lavender gray, yellow, pure white, and powder pink. Color is also a factor to consider in feng shui.

Feng shui, meaning wind-water, is an ancient Chinese practice that focuses on creating harmony between a person and their environment; it is used to create balance and flow. Spruce Environmental Technologies states that it involves "arranging pieces of living space to create balance with the natural world."[141] The website states the four main principles of Feng Shui:

1. **Chi:** Life force energy

2. **Commanding position:** The spot in the room farthest from the door but not directly in line with it. "The commanding position designates where you'll want to spend most of the time in a space. You will want to have a clear line of sight to the door from the commanding position to have the best feng shui possible."

3. **Bagua** (translated as eight-areas): This is a feng shui energy map. "Each area relates to a different life circumstance, such as family, wealth, or career, and each one has corresponding

shapes, colors, seasons, numbers, and earthly elements. At the center of the bagua—a ninth area—is you, representing your overall wellness."

4. **Five elements:** Earth, metal, wind, water, and fire are the elements you want to balance.

An infrared sauna, **sauna bathing**, is linked to relaxation and well-being, stress relief, and improved symptoms of depression and anxiety. A traditional sauna uses heat to warm the air around you, but an infrared sauna uses light to create heat without warming the air around you—making it more tolerable for those who don't like the high heat.

A final practice I have found useful is **Super Brain Yoga**. I used this technique for years as an elementary school teacher and found that it helps children focus and calm down. Super Brain Yoga is a complementary therapy for improving mental health and cognitive function that can reduce anxiety, promote relaxation, and improve physical and mental stability. The short, easy practice involves a series of actions. The Human Condition lists benefits of Super Brain Yoga:

1. Improved academic performance

2. Improved short-term memory

3. Increased academic participation

4. Improved selective attention

5. Improved state and trait mindfulness

6. Improved cognitive function

7. Improved confidence

8. Improved concentration

9. Reductions in state anxiety

10. Improved behavior

11. Greater calm and focus in children with autism

12. Improved focus and social skills in children with ADHD

The Human Condition also gives guidelines on how to perform Super Brain Yoga's 14 steps, plus there are many YouTube videos on the process.[142] I recommend that you learn the steps before following along with the videos so important steps are not missed.

Suggestion: Don't try to do everything discussed; focus on whichever practices resonate with you.

~ VII ~
Final Thoughts

As I reflected on why I wrote this book, it became clear that it is possible to improve depression and anxiety when appropriate steps are taken because, while genetics play a role in our mental health, environment also plays a significant role. According to Stanford Medicine, heritability is only 40% to 50% influential—we can make changes in environmental factors to improve our mental health.[143]

It has also become clear to me that the sooner the mental illness is discovered, the sooner the changes can be made; the National Library of Medicine says about half of all mental disorders start in the mid-teens and about three quarters of all mental disorders start by the mid-twenties.[144]

When we are on the wrong course for our well-being, we increase our likelihood of developing or worsening depression and anxiety. An article by Father Jim Chern, "The Difference One Degree Makes," illustrates this beautifully.[145] Chern explains how a two-degree error in flight coordinates caused a plane to crash into a volcano in 1979. Unfortunately, 257 people died because of this error; the plane was two degrees off for many miles, taking it further and further from the correct destination. The article focused on the negative things that happened to the Pharisees (a strict religious group in Bible times) due to being slightly off God's course. It was a great analogy of what happens to our mental health when we are off course and is why we need to eliminate negative influences in our life and maximize positivity.

I believe that engaging in negative behaviors pushes us off course, a little bit at a time, and eventually we are so off course it is hard to get back on track. This can worsen depression and anxiety and lead to suicidal thinking. In contrast, each positive step we take brings us a degree closer to well-being.

This book has offered many suggestions, but the first step is to see a primary care physician and get a referral to a qualified psychotherapist. Along with counseling, request a full blood workup to rule out any nutritional deficiencies. Also, eat a clean, healthy diet and take any supplements that might be beneficial. Another first step is learning to calm your mind through meditation (transcendental meditation is particularly helpful for PTSD), then incorporating some simpler suggestions, like getting enough sunlight and sleep, and practicing gratitude.

Finally, if you or a person you know seems suicidal, take it seriously and act immediately. In the US, the Suicide & Crisis Lifeline is available for talking or texting at 988. I hope this book will help people have the information needed to positively influence their life and for no other families to endure the loss of someone they love to suicide.

~ VIII ~
The Author's Story

I was born into a family with two parents and two older sisters. I had a happy childhood and was raised in the Lutheran Church. After I graduated from college as a recreation therapist, I got married. It was a difficult marriage because my husband had struggled with depression his entire life. Our first child, Josh, was born 11 days early. I wouldn't have thought this was an issue, but he had respiratory distress syndrome and had to be in the hospital for 11 days. I ended up with a uterine infection and was admitted to a different hospital for several days during this time; it was traumatic because I could not bond with Josh. I remember recording messages to him for his dad to play for Josh so that we could form some sort of bond.

When we got home following our hospitalizations, Josh cried most of the day and night. His doctor told me it was colic, which usually lasts for three months, but Josh had colic for four-and-a-half months. The only way I could calm him at night was to hold him upright and walk around singing. During this time, we became very bonded. Our bond became stronger as he grew, and friends would tell me that we were "super bonded." He did not want anyone else to even hold him.

When Josh was three years old, I decided to put him in preschool. This was such a traumatic experience for Josh. He cried intensely every day when I left but the teacher encouraged me to go quickly. It was one of the most difficult situations that I had to deal with, and it lasted for several months until he finally adjusted. During this time, he had many health problems, including 30+ ear infections. At three, he needed surgery, and then many more surgeries followed that. His brother was born during this time; they were 19 months apart.

Josh started kindergarten at five years old and it was a good experience for him, as his teacher was my sister, his aunt. She taught him phonics and he was successful academically. His youngest brother was born at this time and when Josh went to first grade, he had a miserable year. The focus in education at that time was on "whole language." His teacher did not teach him phonics and because of that he struggled with reading. He was already shy and became insecure of himself academically.

I had happily been a stay-at-home mom, but when Josh was in first grade I went back to work as a recreation therapist for a few hours each afternoon. This was difficult for Josh because I was not there when he got home from school. He started pulling his hair out until I finally quit and decided to stay home again full time. Things got better for him after that for a few years.

When Josh was in fifth grade, I decided I wanted to go into education, so I enrolled in an early childhood education program. After two years, I received my teaching credential and worked in a preschool part-time for about a year then got a job as a kindergarten teacher in 1999 and started working full-time. I worked too many hours as a new teacher and came to regret that. Life was hectic but we made it work. In junior high, Josh started having symptoms of depression, which frequently expresses itself as anger. He went to a counselor, but she said she wasn't making progress with him. He stopped going and his depression got worse. During high school his depression worsened even more. At age 20, he started having suicidal thoughts, and at 21, he took his own life.

When this happened, I didn't know what to do. I struggled with my faith and stopped going to church. I just remember saying over and over, "I don't know what to do." The grief was unimaginable, but I didn't want it to define me; I wanted our family to heal and I knew that was up to me. I told my husband I was not going to stay stuck in grief. This was so clear to me because of my own experiences when I was a young child. My mom's 17-year-old sister died in a car accident and my grandmother never recovered. It had to be very hard on my mom, so when Josh died, I decided that I was not going to do the same thing; and decided that I didn't want my other boys' lives ruined because I could not heal. This led me to find a way to heal. I started going to counseling, which helped immensely. I had so much guilt, but I remember her telling me *If you had known better, you would have done better.* It was true—I didn't have the information to be able to help him. We did a therapy called EMDR (eye movement desensitization and reprocessing) that helped tremendously with the guilt. Another significant event happened during this time; my body hurt terribly, and I was diagnosed with fibromyalgia. The doctor said I needed medication, but I refused it, feeling the diagnosis was ridiculous. So, in my mind, I rejected what I was told and decided I had no pain. It sounds crazy, but that is exactly what happened—to my amazement, the pain dissipated.

While in counseling, I started going to The Oneness Center. This was a New Thought church that taught The Science of Mind principles by Ernest Holmes. I knew nothing about it but when I started going, I felt like I was at home. Their beliefs were completely in line with mine and I started taking helpful classes. I had always believed that we have the power to manifest things in our life by our thinking and based on our subconscious thoughts, which ironically, I learned from my grandmother. She studied under Mary Baker Eddy who developed Christian Science, which was instrumental in the development of Science of Mind.[146] When I didn't feel good or got a cold as a child, she would just say to brush it off our shoulder and it'll go away. It worked. This became abundantly clear during one of my Science of Mind classes.

During one of my first classes when I was just learning how to apply the principles, I discovered how our thoughts create our reality. I challenged the instructor because of some pain I was experiencing. I had bunion surgery many years prior to this that went bad. I ended up having four more surgeries to correct the first surgery. My foot hurt all the time, and I was a teacher, so I was on my feet a lot. I told the instructor that I didn't believe my thoughts and beliefs could make the pain go away (forgetting that my grandmother's words and that I healed myself when diagnosed with fibromyalgia) so she gave me a spiritual mind treatment. I was shocked when one day which I don't remember how long this took, but my foot pain was gone. It made me a true believer in how much power our subconscious thoughts create our reality.

Then in 2011, my husband succumbed to his depression and took his own life. Thankfully, I had my spiritual community, and this helped me work through my pain so much quicker.

I continued to study and take classes on The Science of Mind and in August of 2014, I became a practitioner and learned how to give spiritual mind treatments. At The Oneness Center, I was exposed to many energy practices; I learned Reiki, how to use crystals for healing, meditation, how to use sound to shift energy, and many other practices. I also read many books on shifting our thinking by changing our subconscious thoughts. One of my favorite books, *Handbook to Higher Consciousness*[147] by Ken Keyes, taught me how to change my subconscious mind by memorizing the 12 pathways to higher consciousness. I continued to learn and practice living a more peaceful, happy life. Many people were amazed that I was happy and at peace and I was asked to share my path with our spiritual community at The Oneness Center. I presented my story that explains my path and why I believe shifting energy is critical.

Talk at The Oneness Center, November 30, 2014

I want to share a scene from my favorite movie: *Ghost Busters*. Toward the end of the movie the ghost—Gozer— is about to destroy the Ghost Busters and tells them to choose their destructor. Bill Murray, as Peter Venkman, says, "I get it. Clear your mind." Then Dan Aykroyd, as Ray Stantz, looks guilty and says, "I couldn't help it. It just popped in my head." Next, you see a giant-sized Stay Puft Marshmallow Man who is to be their destructor.

My point: it was Ray's subconscious mind that conjured up the Stay Puft Marshmallow Man. What I want to talk about today is how we can make a conscious effort to not let our subconscious mind determine how we experience life. The iceberg model of consciousness can help us understand what happened. The part of the iceberg visible above the water is about 10%, while most of the iceberg is below the surface (90%). The 10% we see above the water can be thought of as our consciousness, and the 90% that we don't see as our subconsciousness. *Ghost Busters* is the perfect example of that for me because the Stay Puft Marshmallow Man came out of Ray's subconscious mind; he wasn't even aware of it. Therefore, if we don't make a *conscious choice* about what we want to experience, the choice will be made for us from our subconscious mind.

It's up to us to fully utilize the tip of the iceberg, or that 10%; our conscious thoughts. It's that 10% that I want to focus on today. Through our consciousness, we have choice, which I am thankful for. We can choose how we feel depending on what we choose to focus on.

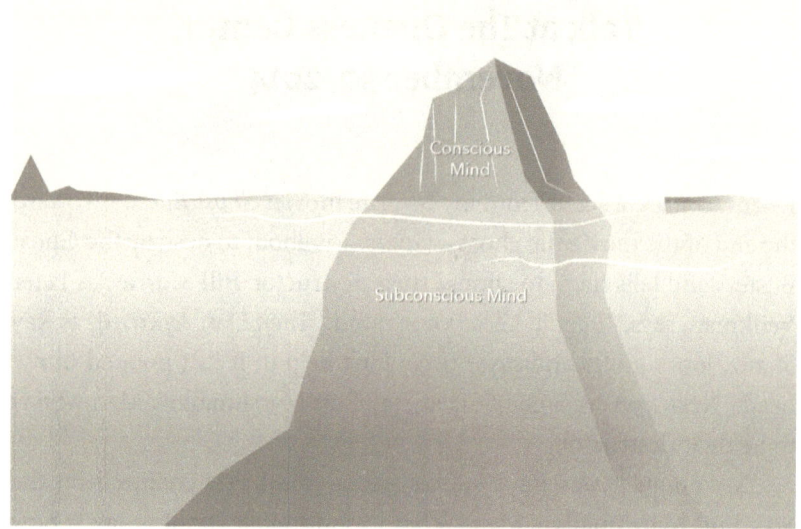

The iceberg theory of consciousness.

Now I want to share my life experiences, and how choice has played such a huge role as far as bringing me peace, joy, and happiness after devastating things that have happened in my life.

First, my childhood. When I was one year old, my mom's 17-year-old sister was killed in a car accident. I experienced the way my grandmother dealt with this loss my entire childhood; she was always crying and sad on holidays and that affected me and the rest of the family. I did not enjoy holidays, and I know it was hard for my mom. I often wondered how that made her feel when she was still living but her mom was grieving for her sister.

Fast forward many years, I got married and had three boys. My oldest son struggled with depression and anxiety his entire life, and at 21 years of age, he took his own life. Strangely, amid my pain, I decided that I was not going to let this destroy me or my two other boys. I remembered how painful it was to watch my grandmother suffer and I made a choice almost immediately that I was not going to do that to my boys even though I was so devastated by the loss of Josh that

I could barely function. My anxiety was out of control; I had to take antianxiety medication just to get through the day. I had to take many drugs just to sleep—which was all I wanted to do. Sleep. I was taking Ativan, two Tylenol PM, and two Ambien sleeping pills just to fall asleep. My body hurt all the time, and I was soon diagnosed with fibromyalgia. I rejected this diagnosis, and it disappeared completely. The only thing that brough me comfort was reading books on the afterlife and medium communication. As I wandered bookstores, I saw books on spirituality and started reading those: Gary Zukav,[148] Eckhart Tolle,[149] Wayne Dyer,[150] Louise Hay,[151] and many others and that gave me a sense of peace, which I was so desperately looking for.

Then I learned about The Oneness Center, a New Thought community, and decided to go to a Sunday service. I knew immediately that I had found my home and started attending regularly. It wasn't long before I started taking Science of Mind classes that taught me about our conscious and subconscious mind. I also started getting affirmative prayer, Spiritual Mind Treatments, from one of the ministers for pain. To my amazement, my pain pretty much disappeared. So, I continued to study, took class after class, and started learning how to apply these principles in my own life.

Then my husband, who had cancer and never dealt effectively with our son's death, took his own life. Well, as you can imagine, I was totally devastated again. I went back into depression and anxiety. My only comfort was food, and I gained 35 pounds. Fortunately, I had The Oneness Center, and I consciously chose to continue attending classes and applying the principles I was learning.

Then I took a class called "The Power of Decision," and this completely changed my life.[152] During this class, I realized that the decision was mine: I could let my subconscious continue to rule over me and be depressed and anxious, or I could make a conscious choice to change my thinking. I chose to change my thinking. I decided that night that I wanted peace, joy, and happiness again. What is amazing is that once we make a conscious choice, the universe (God) aligns with that energy and changes occur. Once I made that decision, I put some effort into making changes in my life. I decided that I needed to get out and have some fun, so I joined a bowling league. This led to making new friends, becoming more active socially, and doing more things that got me out of my house and feeling sorry for myself. Since that original decision, I have made an amazing shift in my life. I do not struggle with anxiety or depression anymore and I lost the 35 pounds. I have the inner peace that I was longing for and I'm happier now than I have ever been.

For me, it all came down to that choice that I made within myself. I decided that I wanted peace, joy, and happiness, and the universe (God) aligned with that vibration, and that is what I have now. In *The Science of Mind*,[153] Ernest Holmes says, "We cannot live a choiceless life. Every day, every moment, every second, there is a choice. If it were not so, we would not be individuals. We have the right to choose what we wish to experience." As for me, I choose peace, joy, and happiness. And I leave you with one question: What are you choosing for your life?

I believe that because I changed my subconscious mind and I was finally at peace and happy, I met my current husband, and we were married in 2018. While I have continued to practice Science of Mind principles, we have also started attending a local Lutheran Church and became members. I retired from teaching in 2023, and I now have time to focus on sharing the research I have done over the years on prevention of suicide.

(Some content was removed because it is not relevant to this book.)

~ IX ~
Resources

Suicideispreventable.org

https://www.my.clevelandclinic.org/health/articles/suicide

988lifeline.org

https://www.suicideispreventable.org

Crisistexline.org: 741741

https://qprinstitute.com

Veteranscrisisline.net

Thetrevorproject.org

Lgbthotline.org

Athletehelpline.org

Samaritanhope.org

Nami.org

Lgbecomingout.org

Theyouthline.org

Teenlineonline.org

Nationalsafeplace.org

Samhsa.gov

Nationalparentyouthhelpline.org

Gradresources.org

Centerstone.org

Blackline.com

Physiciansupportline.com

Healthyamericas.org

~ X ~
# References

II. Warning Signs of Suicide and Resources

1 https://my.clevelandclinic.org/health/articles/suicide
2 https://www.iasp.info/
3 https://www.crisistextline.org/
4 https://qprinstitute.com/

IV. Mind

5 Dyer, Wayne W. *You'll See It When You Believe It.* HarperCollins Publishing Inc., 2001
6 Lipton, Bruce H. *The Biology of Belief.* Hay House, Inc. 2005.

1. Psychological Counseling (Psychotherapy)

7   Cromwell, Kathy. CT, MSW, LCSW. 2024
8   https://www.mayoclinic.org
9   https://www.apa.org
10 https://www.emdr.com/
11 https://my.clevelandclinic.org/health/treatments/22838 -dialectical-behavior-therapy-dbt
12 https://www.apa.org/topics/anxiety/disorders
13 https://my.clevelandclinic.org/health/treatments/22676-hypnosis

2. Treatment-Resistant Depression

14 https://www.hopkinsmedicine.org/health/conditions-and
-diseases/mood-disorders/treatment-resistant-depression

15 https://pmc.ncbi.nlm.nih.gov/articles/PMC10503923/

16 https://www.mayoclinic.org/diseases-conditions/depression
/in-depth/treatment-resistant-depression/art-20044324

17 https://my.clevelandclinic.org/health/treatments/17507-stellate
-ganglion-block

18 https://www.jasonattaman.com>painblog ...
https://jasonattaman.com/pain-blog/

19 https://www.amenclinics.com

20 changeyourbrain.org

4. Gratitude

21 Smith, Ashley J. "Gratitude—A Mental Health Game Changer."
Anxiety & Depression Association of America.

22 https://greatergood.berkeley.edu/article/item/how_gratitude
_changes_you_and_your_brain

23 Byrne, Rhonda. *The Magic.* Atria Books, 2012.

24 https://www.mindful.org/an/introduction/to/mindful/gratitude

25 https://www.calm.com

26 Hawkins, David R. *Power vs Force.* Hay House Inc., 2012.

27 https://www.facebook.com/drwaynedyer/posts/if-you-have
-a-choice-between-being-right-or-being-kind-choose-kind
-drwayne-dyer/10153727856701030/

28 https://self-compassion.org>self-compassion-practices

29 https://www.mentalhealth.org.uk/explore-mental-health
/kindness/kindness-matters-guide

30 Emoto, Masaru. *The Hidden Messages in Water.* Beyond Words
Publishing, Inc., 2004.

31 https://timesofindia.indiatimes.com

32 https://pmc.ncbi.nlm.nih.gov/articles/PMC3000745/

33 https://marquemedical.com/effects-of-negativity/
34 Holmes, Ernest. The Science of Mind. Putnam Books, 1938.

7. Positive Self-Affirmations

35 Wellspringprevention.org
36 Hay, Louise L. You Can Heal Your Life. Hay House, Inc., 1999.
37 Wellspringprevention.org
38 Byrne, Rhonda. The Secret. Atria Books, 2006.
39 Wilde, Stuart. Miracles. Hay House, Inc., 2007.
40 Dyer, Wayne W. You'll See It When You Believe It. HarperCollins Publishing, Inc., 2001.
41 Bernstein, Gabrielle. Super Attractor. Hay House, LLC, 2021.
42 Freeman, Janet Marie. I Am Source Code. 2019.

8. Forgiveness

43 Greatergood.berkeley.edu/topic/forgiveness/definition
44 https://www.verywellmind.com
45 https://www.mayoclinic.org/healthy-lifestyle/adult-health/in-depth/forgiveness/art-20047692

9. Pharmaceuticals

46 Journal of American Medicine Association, September 12, 2023 issue
47 https://www.skipsimpson.com>suicide>medications-with-suicide-risks
48 https://vox.com/science-and-health/2018/6/14/17458726/depression-drugssuicide-sideeffects
49 https://www.amenclinics.com
50 https://www.ncbi.nlm.nih.gov>books>NBK361016
51 https://www.hopkinsmedicine.org/health/conditions-and-diseases/mooddisorders/treatment-resistant-depression

10. Social Media

52 https://www.vantagefit.io

53 https://www.hhs.gov/sites/default/files/sg-youth-mental-health
-socialmedia-summary

54 https://news.gallup.com/poll/512576/teens-spend-average-hours
-social-media-per-day.aspx

11. Watching the News and Television

55 https://www.psychiatrist.com

56 https://www.health.harvard.edu/mind-and-mood/too-much-tv-
might-be-bad-for-your-brain

57 "Protecting Our Mental Health from Negative News Coverage."
Johns Hopkins University and Medicine https://hr.jhu.edu
/wp-content/uploads/JHEAP_Negative-News-Coverage-and
-Mental-Health.pdf

58 https://www.amenclinics.com

59 https://www.aa.org

60 https://americanaddictioncenters.org

61 https://salvationarmyusa.ort>usn>rehabilitation

62 https://recovery.com>condition>alcohol

63 https://findtreatment.gov

64 https://www.samsha.gov>offices-centers>cast

V. Introduction: Body
13. Nutrition

65 Watts, Martina. Nutrition and Mental Health: A Handbook.
Pavilion Publishing and Media, Ltd., 2008

66 https://www.verywellhealth.com

67 Kaplan, Bonnie J, and Julia J. Rucklidge. The Better Brain:
Overcome Anxiety, Combat Depression, and Reduce ADHA and
Stress with Nutrition. Houghton Mifflin Harcourt Publishing
Company, 2021.

68 www.truehope.com
69 https://hardynutritionals.com/

14. Supplements

70 https://www.mayoclinic.org/diseases-conditions/depression
    /expertanswer/natural-remedies-for-depression/faq20058026
71 https://www.jeffersonhealth.org/your-health/living-well
    /8supplements-thatcan-help-reduce-anxiety-according-to-a-psych
72 https://doi.org/10.3390/ijms24087098

15. Sleep

73 https://www.hopkinsmedicine.org/health/wellness-and-prevention
    /depression-and-sleep-understanding-the-connection
74 https://www.health.harvard.edu/newsletter_article/8-secrets
    -to-a-good-nights-sleep
75 https://neurology.weill.cornell.edu/about-us/videos
76 https://www.mayoclinic.org/healthy-lifestyle/adult-health/in-depth
    /napping/art-20048319#:~:text=For%20most%20people%2C%20
    short%20naps,might%20interfere%20with%20nighttime%20sleep.

16. Water

77 https://drinkoptimum.com
78 https://www.cnet.com
79 https://www.umsystem.edu/totalrewards/wellness/how-to
    -calculate-how-much-water-you-should-drink#:~:text
    =The%20good%20news%20is%20there,program%20for%
    20faculty%20and%20staff
80 https://www.frizzlife.com/blogs/news/does-alkaline-water-help
    -with-anxiety?srsltid=AfmBOopqw6jrDywgQ5Gqlv6YmuOKbd
    E6d-jR3b8Ep3AUhrCMrNqpRnlI
81 https://www.mayoclinichealthsystem.org/hometown-health
    /speaking-of-health/tips-for-drinking-more-water

17. Grounding

82 Raypole, Crystal. "30 Grounding Techniques to Quiet Distressing Thoughts." https://www.healthline.com/health/grounding -techniques

18. Exercise and Movement

83 https://www.mayoclinic.org/diseases-conditions/depression /in-depth/depression-and-exercise/art-20046495

84 https://www.mentalhealth.org.uk/our-work/public-engagement /mental-health-awareness-week/movement-research#:~:text =Exercise%20releases%20%E2%80%9Cfeel%20good%E2%80%9 D%20hormones,also%20boost%20our%20mental%20health

19. Yoga

85 https://aurawellnesscenter.com

86 https://www.health.harvard.edu/mind-and-mood/exercise-is -an-all-natural-treatment-to-fight-depression#:~:text =One%20in%2010%20adults%20in,helps%20regulate%20 mood%E2%80%94is%20smaller

20. Massage Therapy

87 https://www.mayoclinic.org/tests-procedures/massage-therapy /about/pac-20384595#:~:text=The%20soft%20tissues%20include %20muscle,offer%20it%20with%20standard%20treatment.

88 https://www.nuhs.edu/4-mental-benefits-of-massage-therapy/

21. Chiropractic Therapy

89 https://aica.com/does-chiropractic-care-help-with-anxiety -and-depression/

90 https://anchortohealth.com/2022/02/25/3-reasons-you-should -choose-neurological-based-chiropractic-care/

91 https://doi.org/10.15412/J.BCN.03070208

22. Traditional Chinese Medicine (TCM)

92 https://www.verywellmind.com/chinese-medicine-8649196

93 https://www.nccih.nih.gov/health/traditional-chinese-medicine
-what-you-need-to-know

94 https://muih.edu/using-chinese-medicine-for-treating-depression
-and-anxiety/

95 https://doi.org/10.1155/2022/1442578

24. Acupuncture, Acupressure, and Emotional Freedom Technique

96 https://www.nuhs.edu/why-psychiatrists-are-recommending
-acupuncture-to-their-patients/

97 https://www.healthline.com/health/eft-tapping

VI. Introduction: Spirit

98 https://www.dictionary.com/browse/soul

99 https://www.mcleanhospital.org/essential/spirituality

25. Energy

100 Byrne, Rhonda. The Secret. Atria Books, 2006.

101 Hawkins, David R. Power vs Force. Hay House, Inc., 2012.

26. Prayer

102 https://www.psychologytoday.com/us/blog/talking-about-men
/201912/prayer-and-mental-health

103 https://www.biblestudytools.com/topical-verses/healing
-bible-verses/

104 https://dornsife.usc.edu/news/stories/what-is-a-miracle/

105 https://give.stellmarisfamily.org/news/mother-teresas-favorite
-prayer

106 Holmes, Ernest. Science of Mind. Putnam books, 1938.

27. Meditation

107 https://www.un.org/en/observances/meditation-day

108 https://www.massgeneral.org/charged/episodes/sara-lazar

109 https://www.healthline.com/nutrition/12-benefits-of-meditation

110 Ywyman, James F. The Moses code. Hay House, LLC., 2021.

111 https://psych-k.com

112 Dyer, Wayne W. Meditations for Manifestation. Audio CD, 2004.

113 https://insighttimer.com

114 https://www.nhs.uk/every-mind-matters/mental-wellbeing-tips
/how-to-meditate-for-beginners/#7-steps

115 https://www.gonoodle.com

116 https://www.healthychildren.org

117 https://live.meditateamerica.org

118 https://www.tm.org/blog/stress-benefits

119 https://www.davidlynchfoundation.org.uk/about-tm.html

28. Music

120 https://pubmed.ncbi.nlm.nih.gov/9439023/

121 https://www.merriam-webster.com/dictionary/grunge

29. Vibrational Sound Therapy

122 https://www.academyofsoundhealing.com

123 https://astutecounseling.com

124 https://www.rush.edu/news/what-vibrational-sound-therapy

125 Spiritseekerhealing.com/vibrational-sound-therapy

126 https://reikihealingassociation.com/reiki-for-mental-wellbeing
-supporting-your-mind-with-reiki-energy/

31. Crystal Healing

127 https://theenergyflows.com

128 Permutt, Philip. The Crystal Healer. CICO Books, 2007.

32. Laughter

129 https://www.scientificamerican.com/article/a-healthy-laugh

130 https://www.ucl.ac.uk/icn/prople/sophie-scott

131 McGhee, Paul. Human as Survival Training for a Stressed-Out World: The 7 Habits Program. AuthorHouse, 2010.

132 https://www.laughteryoga.org

33. Nature

133 Qing, Li. Forest Bathing: How Trees Can Help You Find Health and Happiness. Penguin Life, 2018.

134 https://time.com/collection/guide-to-happiness/4306455/stress-relief-nature/

135 https://www.fs.usda.gov/about-agency/features/healing-power-nature

34. Sunshine

136 https://www.healthline.com/health/seasonal-affective-disorder

35. Animals

137 https://www.findhelp.org

138 https://www.assistancedog.center

139 https://www.southnavotoanimalhospital.com

36. Additional Ways to Raise Your Vibration

140 https://www.spiritandmuse.com

141 https://www.thespruce.com

142 Thehumancondition.com/superbrain-yoga

VII. Final Thoughts

143 https://med.stanford.edu/depressiongenetics/mddandgenes.html

144 pubmed.ncbi.nlm.nih.gov/17551351/

145 https://homilyonthespot.com

VIII. The Author's Story

146 Eddy, Mary Baker. Science and Health with Key to the Scriptures. The Christian Science Publishing Society, 1917.

147 Keyes, Ken, Jr. Handbook to Higher Consciousness. Living Love Publications, 1979.

148 garyzukav@seatofthesoul.com

149 Tolle, Eckhart. The Power of Now. Namaste Publishing, 1997.

150 Dyer, Wayne W. I Can See Clearly Now. Hay House, Inc., 2014.

151 Hay, Louise L. You Can Heal Your Life. Hay House, Inc., 1999.

152 Barker, Raymond Charles. The Power of Decision. Penguin Group, 1988.

153 Holmes, Ernest. The Science of Mind. Putnam Books, 1938.

Acknowledgments

I would like to express gratitude for all the support and encouragement I have received throughout this journey from my husband, Larry, my sons Justin and Jordan, and my friends Mina Borders and Jackie Taggart. I am also grateful to beta readers Jackie Taggart, Judy Drilling, Janette Freeman, and Jessica Garcia for giving me valuable feedback to improve this book. I am sincerely grateful to the people who spent time answering my questions and giving me valuable information in their area of expertise: Cathy Abeyta, Jessica Garcia, Crissy Campbell, Judy Drilling, and Kathy Cromwell. I am also grateful to my editor, Heather Pendley, and to Carla Green for formatting and designing the book. Last, this book could not have been written if it were not for all the synchronicities that occurred while writing it, and for this, I give gratitude to God.

About the Author

Suzanne Oliver is a mother of three sons. One lives abroad, one lives in northern California, and one lives in the spirit realm—Josh. Losing Josh to suicide in 2007 was one of the hardest experiences imaginable for Suzanne. It was also a time of great reflection, which led Suzanne to the conclusion that more information on suicide prevention needed to be readily available to the public. From then on, anytime she heard of new research in suicide prevention, she would put it in her folder, with the intention that one day she would be able to share that information with those struggling with mental health issues. Then, in 2011, her husband, who blamed himself for Josh's depression and anxiety, also took his own life.

During her time of self-reflection, Suzanne was introduced to a Religious Science church and discovered many practices for improving her mental health. She benefited from these practices so much that she studied and became a practitioner. She is also trained in several other healing practices, including Reiki.

She began her career as a Recreational Therapist and worked with individuals with mental illness, among other disabilities. Once she started her family, she was a stay-at-home mom until her sons were in school full time. At that time, she received her early childhood teaching credential and taught elementary school for 25 years.

Since retiring in 2023, she has devoted her time to researching how to help individuals with anxiety, depression, and suicidal thinking. Her mission is to make this information readily available for those who need it. She also believes that children need to learn how to take care of their mental health at an early age. That is why she is publishing a children's book next year, based on the holistic strategies discussed in *Right Now!*

Suzanne remarried in 2018 and lives in Fresno, California, with her husband Larry and cat, Boomer. She enjoys spending time with family and friends, traveling, reading, and spending time in her beautiful backyard, especially in the summer.

Coming Soon

Children's book—This is a fun, colorful, interactive book for elementary school children, teaching them the strategies introduced in this book in a way that they can relate to. Includes information for parents and teachers on how to use the strategies effectively. Will be available in 2026.

Science fiction book—This is based on the future, when we live in an almost peaceful world. Most people have evolved into a kind, loving, place in which they focus on their well-being, but there are certain groups of people who have not evolved, and this leads to occasional problems. The story is centered around one of my descendants, who—like me—has three children, and must figure out how to help one of her children. Will be available in 2027.